BROTHERS IN ARMS

CANADIAN FIREFIGHTERS IN ENGLAND IN THE SECOND WORLD WAR

JOHN LEETE & BRIAN BERRINGER

AMBERLEY

First published 2015

Amberley Publishing
The Hill, Stroud, Gloucestershire, GL5 4EP
www.amberley-books.com

Copyright © John Leete and Brian Berringer, 2015

The right of John Leete and Brian Berringer to be identified as the Author of
this work has been asserted in accordance with the Copyrights, Designs and
Patents Act 1988.

ISBN 978 1 4456 4825 5 (print)
ISBN 978 1 4456 4826 2 (ebook)

British Library Cataloguing in Publication Data.
A catalogue record for this book is available from the British Library.

Typesetting by Amberley Publishing.
Printed in the UK.

CONTENTS

Foreword   4

Preface   10

1   Take Cover   15

2   Defending the Home Front   18

3   A Measure of National Importance   23

4   Active Defences   42

5   All for One and One for All   62

6   Brothers in Arms   84

    Epilogue   104

    The Eternal Flame   107

    Acknowledgements   127

FOREWORD

I am delighted that an unusual historical fact and important part of the overall story of the role of the fire service during the Second World War, is now being explained in this book. It is dedicated to those who volunteered to form 'The Corps of (Civilian) Canadian Firefighters' and who then came to England in support of the National Fire Service (NFS).

In July 1941, the Canadian Government decided to send a contingent of firefighters to the United Kingdom to assist in dealing with the many and large fires caused by the Nazi air raids on our nation's cities and towns. Volunteers were recruited from various locations in Canada and were brought together in Ottawa for initial training and equipping.

The first contingent arrived in Britain by sea on 24 June 1942 as part of an Atlantic convoy, a perilous journey in itself with the continuous threat of attack by submarines.

Following a welcome ceremony in London on 30 June, the Corps were split and sent to two separate training locations. Those destined to serve in Southampton and Portsmouth were sent to the NFS No. 6 (Southern) Training School located at Testwood School in Totton, near Southampton and those destined

to serve in Bristol and Plymouth were sent to the NFS No. 7 (South Western) School at Lee Mill, Ivybridge, near Plymouth.

On completion of training and the issue of vehicles and equipment, the men were sent to their stations and placed on active duty as part of the NFS. They crewed NFS issued vehicles, but were easily identified by the different style of their Canadian-issue uniform. A small administrative group was also detached to London, but did not perform active firefighting duties.

In addition to fighting fires in Southampton, Portsmouth, Plymouth and Bristol, they took part in deployments of reinforcement to other cities and towns suffering air attack. They were also involved with the various fire service operations associated with the build-up of the allied armed forces and their equipment, in preparation for the D-Day landings. A volunteer detachment of the Corps also trained at Testwood School, as part of 'No. 6 Column of the NFS Overseas Contingent', established to follow closely behind advancing troops as they progressed the liberation of Europe.

Their return home to Canada commenced on 16 December 1944 and the last contingent left the shores of the United

Kingdom on 19 August 1945, some with new brides. Ultimately 406 Canadians came to Britain. Sadly, three of those volunteers lost their lives while deployed.

This remains the largest international deployment of firefighters ever to have taken place, playing a major part in the 'Home Front' and the defence of the United Kingdom.

The contribution made by these volunteers, in support of the men and women of the fire service of the United Kingdom, who had been very much in the 'front line' of the civilian population as a result of bombing raids and, later, attack by 'flying bombs' and rockets, should never be forgotten.

Dave Curry
Chief Officer
Hampshire Fire and Rescue Service

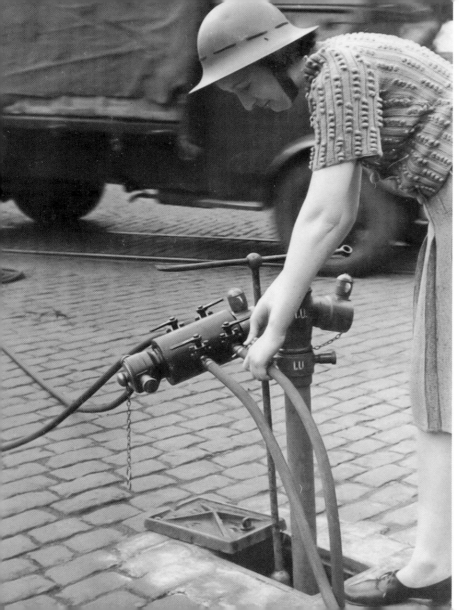

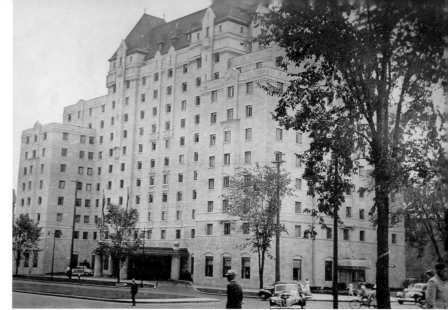

Above: Ottawa, *c.*1941.

Left: A member of what was known as a street firefighting party.

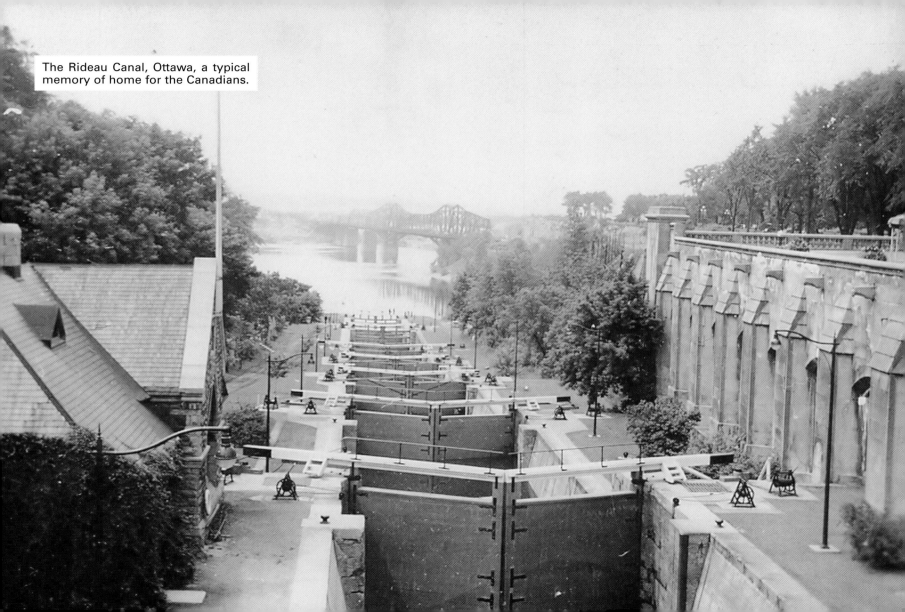

The Rideau Canal, Ottawa, a typical memory of home for the Canadians.

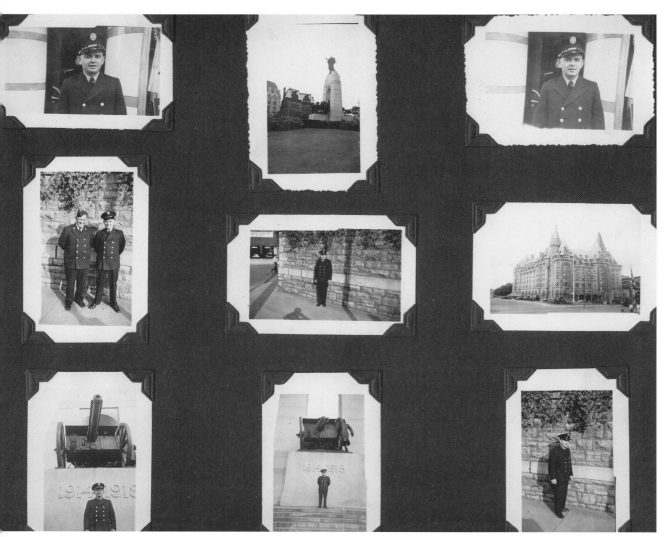

Personal photos
Above: Nine polyphotos taken by a Corps member before leaving Canada: two firemen are shown at sites around Ottawa.

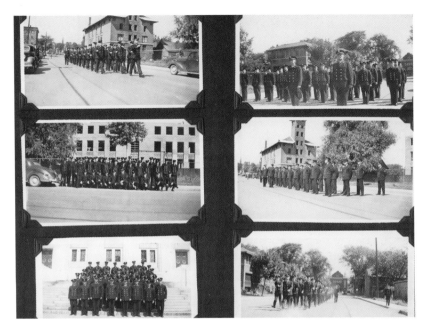

A Further Selection of Personal Photographs
Right: Members of the Corps were able to take photographs, as there appeared to be no problems regarding the supply of film.

Leaving Home
Left: Just before leaving Canada, several parades took place in Ottawa. These photographs show various members of the Corps.

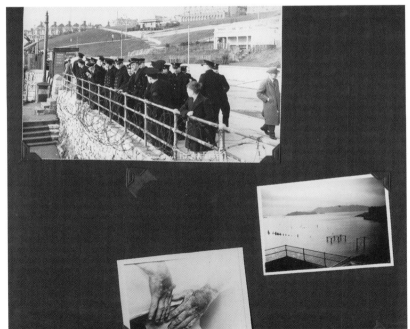

PREFACE

The Fire Services in the United Kingdom are organised to serve urban and rural communities as part of a tried and tested local authority structure with roots dating back to the 1940s.

Yet, before the outbreak of the Second World War, such services, where they existed, were lacking in any real cohesion and in fact, before the implementation of the Fire Brigades Act of 1938, brigades were organised by various independent and commercial bodies which had few legal obligations or controls to meet.

This story begins in 1937, at a time when many people still believed that the political issues in central Europe could be resolved without the need for any conflict. Some in government and commerce, though, had already been making contingencies should war come.

Internationally in 1937, Amelia Earhart, the pioneering aviator, vanished without trace. Walt Disney introduced *Snow White and the Seven Dwarfs*, considered to be a film masterpiece of its time. The German airship *Hindenburg* crashed in flames. Closer to home, idealists were flocking to Spain to fight in the civil war, Egypt became the fifty-ninth member of the League of Nations and Reims Cathedral was reopened following its twenty-year restoration after the First World War.

In Britain, the government's plan to treble the strength of the Royal Air Force, was completed, but in contrast, the chancellor, Neville Chamberlain, was warning that the arms budget was far too low. In the spring of 1937, the aircraft carrier *Ark Royal* was launched and in November MPs voted in favour of a plan that called for air raid shelters to be built in centres of population across the country.

There was some opposition to this proposal, yet Winston Churchill said that air raid shelters were indispensable and that 'well-organised precautions' would mean that any future air attacks on Britain would not be worthwhile – because they would have little impact upon the population. The government subsequently introduced the Air Raid Precautions (ARP) Act in what was regarded as a tangible demonstration of preparations for war.

This act had a direct impact on the nation's fragmented fire service. The act placed responsibilities on rural, district and borough councils to make preparations for dealing with fires caused by air raids. As a result, the Auxiliary Fire Service (AFS) as a new and separate organisation under the direction of local chief officers was created. There were also many privately and commercially operated fire brigades at this time and in some Metropolitan districts of the country, the police were responsible for provision of the brigades and for firefighting.

Just as the reorganisation of the brigades began, the prospect of war in Europe became inevitable. Within a year of the outbreak of war, the government put out a call to the Commonwealth for firefighters to assist in dealing with the onslaught of air raids upon Britain. Later, in 1941, the National Fire Service (NFS) evolved as a more cohesive organisation, which not only absorbed the various disparate services, but also drew upon the lessons learned and experience gained during the early years of the war. The NFS was better able to deal with the challenges then facing the country not least because of improved communications and resources.

However, the history of Britain's Fire Service during the Second World War would not be complete without the inclusion of the little-known story of the volunteer Canadian firefighters who travelled to England to assist the NFS with both firefighting and rescue work until war's end in 1945.

In response to the appeal in 1940 from the British government to Commonwealth countries for up to a thousand men to work alongside our hard-pressed fire services in blitzed towns and cities, it was Canada that quickly responded to the call. However, while research suggests that unforeseen practical and political challenges meant that the first contingents of Canadians did not arrive in England until two years later, it also suggests that these challenges could have been addressed and overcome very quickly if there had been the will by both governments to do so.

The first draft of the Corps arrived in London on 30 June 1942 and was officially recognised on behalf of the British government by the Honourable Herbert Morrison, Minister of National War Services, in the following address.

Please convey to the Canadian Government our thanks and appreciation of this practicable gesture, which is a source of energy and strength to all ranks of the National Fire Service. Your firemen will now take their place along with your soldiers and airmen already here at the side of their British comrades.

The Corps was unique in that, for the first time in history, professional firefighters had left their own country and volunteered to operate, in their own profession, in a theatre of war.

The Corps of Canadian Firefighters, also known as the Canadian Corps of Firefighters, arrived by ship in Liverpool from where they travelled to NFS training schools in Totton, Hampshire, which was an NFS training school. Here they learnt techniques about firefighting in wartime and here too they learnt, in a very short time, much about the English way of life.

After training, contingents were dispatched to Plymouth, Bristol, Portsmouth and Bristol, and the Headquarters Unit was accommodated in Wimbledon, London.

The story of the Canadian firefighters is based upon original research and work by John Leete. Now, with additional material from Brian Berringer and the inclusion of over a hundred rare original images of the Canadians taken before departing their homeland and during their service in England, the story is complete. This unique photographic collection was recorded by one of the wartime Canadian firefighters, and it serves to add great depth and significance to a unique story.

The photographs are exclusive to this book and are published as a complete set for the first time.

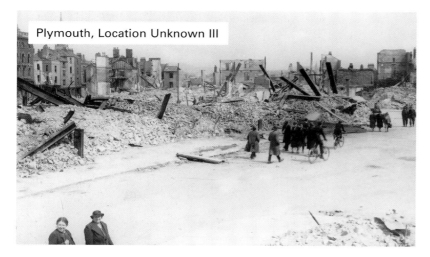

Plymouth, Location Unknown III

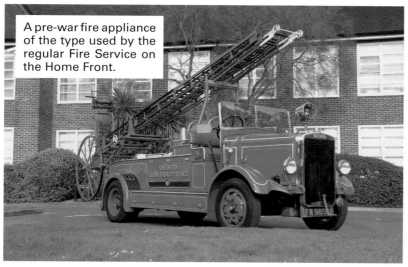

A pre-war fire appliance of the type used by the regular Fire Service on the Home Front.

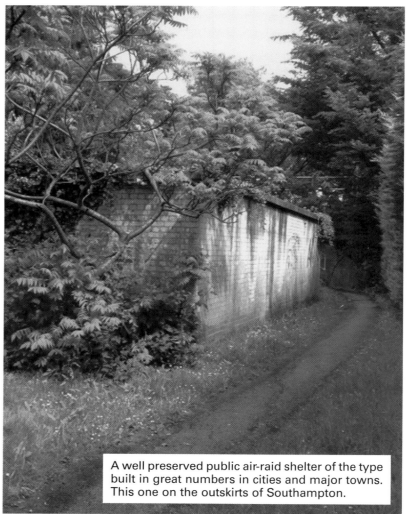

A well preserved public air-raid shelter of the type built in great numbers in cities and major towns. This one on the outskirts of Southampton.

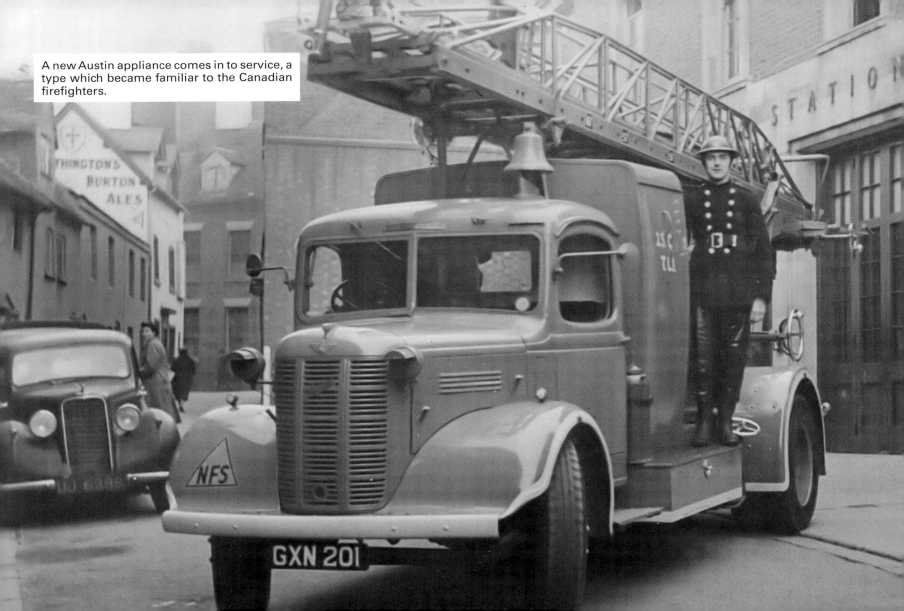

A new Austin appliance comes in to service, a type which became familiar to the Canadian firefighters.

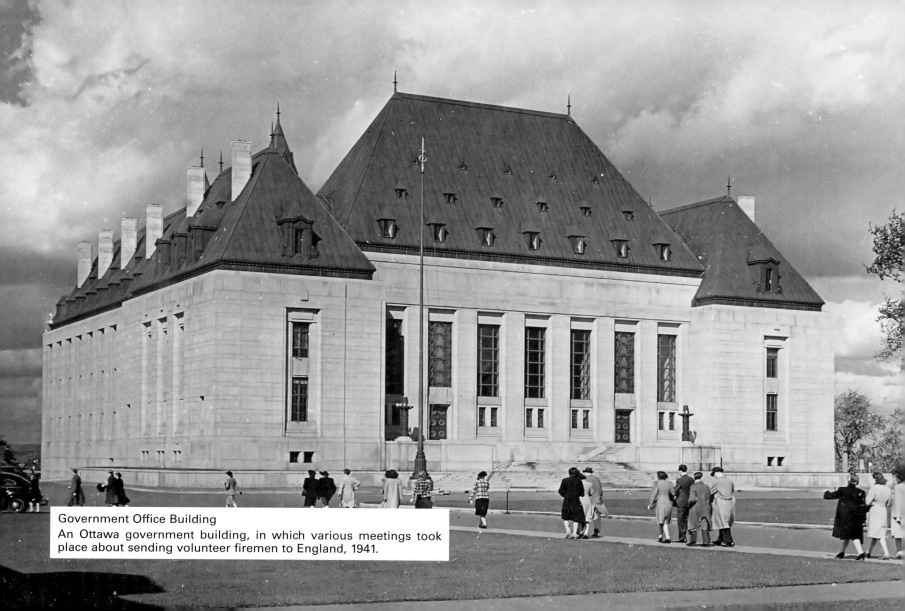

Government Office Building
An Ottawa government building, in which various meetings took place about sending volunteer firemen to England, 1941.

1

TAKE COVER

On 24 December 1914, a lone German aeroplane dropped a bomb near Dover Castle on the south-east coast in Kent. No real damage was to result although, not surprisingly, windows in the area were shattered and there was widespread public panic and concern. Politicians expressed concern at this somewhat unexpected turn of events. This was the first air attack by enemy aircraft on British soil.

Five months later, at the end of May 1915, over a ton of bombs were discharged over London by a German airship. In this single concentrated attack over thirty people were injured and it is recorded that seven people lost their lives. Yet it was not just major cities such as London that suffered the onslaught of enemy bombing. Later during that same year, in the small community of Woodbridge in Suffolk, some ten miles inland on the east coast, twenty-eight bombs were dropped. This resulted in six fatalities in the Cumberland Street area of the town.

David Barney says that his grandmother told him,

During the Great War everyone ran out to watch the first Zeppelin attack on London. We could see the crew who dropped the bombs from the gondola as the searchlights lit up the huge gas bag. A cheer went up from the streets when the hydrogen gas bag exploded with a roar of flames after being hit from ground fire, but then it all fell silent as the crowd watched the crew fall to earth.

For the next eight months, night attacks by Zeppelin airships on Britain were frequent, and it was quite a while before effective counter-measures were devised and implemented by home security. Although London was the usual target, many factors, including the difficulties of basic navigation, resulted in the enemy's craft wandering over the countryside, dropping bombs on villages and towns and causing considerable damage as well as panic among the populace. One example of such panic occurred in Hull, where locals ransacked shops apparently owned by Germans. After a raid on the town in June 1915, twenty-four people lay dead and many more were injured. More than forty properties were destroyed during the raid. Riots broke out, and it was only after the intervention of the army that calm was restored, although feelings of anger and hatred lingered long.

The last deliberate airship raid recorded was in January 1916, and occurred over the industrial heartland of the Midlands.

However, by this time the losses of Zeppelins as a result of more effective defence measures employed on the Home Front, was sufficient to force the Germans to discontinue the use of airships as bombing platforms against Britain. The subsequent introduction of Gotha's twin-engine assault aircraft stepped up the bombing campaign to an unprecedented level. Severe raids on London in June 1917 by fourteen such aircraft resulted in the deaths of over 150 people and injuries to many hundreds of civilians, and a few weeks later there were further casualties sustained in a similar raid. The passions of the general public were now stirred, and there was widespread indignation against the enemy and considerable concern expressed about the effectiveness of the country's defences. Interestingly, the outcome of these events was to prompt the War Cabinet into appointing a special adviser on home defence, one General Jan Smuts. His reports to the Cabinet on matters of home defence and related issues were to directly and positively influence the decision to create the Royal Air Force from the RFC (Royal Flying Corps) in April 1918.

In 1917, the public had grown war-weary and were calling for 'necessary change' on the Home Front. The introduction of proper warnings of air raids and the widespread introduction of public shelters were high on the list of such change. Of course this was against the background of stories of possible gas attacks on the population, further exacerbated by nervousness at the apparent inability of the country to defend itself. Remember, the popular belief was that the war, which began in August 1914, would be over by Christmas of the same year. Few had imagined that it would last for more than a handful of months; and so by the third year with little end in sight it was inevitable that the public would expect more in the way of protection.

It was not until the summer of 1917 that the government, seemingly in reluctant mood, gave in to public concern by providing a rudimentary system of air raid warnings in London. The warnings devised were as basic as they were fairly ineffective, and consisted for the most part of the use of policemen on foot, on bicycles and in cars. Whistles would be blown, horns sounded and placards bearing the words 'Take Cover' would be waved furiously. Limited use of maroons (or sound bombs) was also authorised. The matter of public shelters was similarly met with some indifference, and it was only tempered by the fact that the Commissioner of Police for London gave permission for the use of police stations as public shelters. For some time the public had been using the Underground as a place of refuge although gradually, widespread use of basements in a range of public buildings became an acceptable and recognised practice. In the provinces, such matters as shelter provision was left to the local authorities and considerable work was undertaken in this regard, including the adaption of caves and mine workings in areas where those facilities existed.

The War Cabinet had previously discussed the possibility of large-scale air attacks on London by many aircraft and the likelihood of huge fires being started on a scale that was well beyond the capacity of the fire brigades. They also considered the advantages of taking widespread anti-gas precautions. However, these discussions took place at a time when the ebb and flow of the war was moving in the favour of the Allies. The last attack on London was on 20 May 1918, and this was also to be the last air attack on Britain during the First World War.

Many lessons were learnt and many new experiences befell the population, in particular people being killed in their own homes in a country that had not been occupied by an enemy. The government was finally prepared to recognise that the passive defence of the country, particularly in terms of air raid precautions, civil defence and firefighting, was of great importance from a military point of view. They had already seen for themselves the movement of men and equipment from other vital work to Home Air Defence activities.

They also recognised that, to an enemy, the advantages of air attack could be justified purely on the grounds of the damage, disruption and crippling effect it could have on a civilian population. During the First World War, the Germans dropped about 300 tons of bombs on Britain. In a subsequent war, greater capacities could be dropped from fleets of aircraft, or so a hypothetical study of possible future air attacks concluded. In 1923, at a meeting of the Committee on the Co-ordination of Departmental Action on the Outbreak of War (CCDAOW), the Air Ministry recommended that the Home Office was the relevant department to organise civil defence and to create an air raid precautions scheme. This decision was subsequently endorsed in 1924 by Ramsay MacDonald's Labour government.

2

DEFENDING THE HOME FRONT

The committee which evolved from the meeting of CCDAOW in 1922 held its own inaugural meeting on 15 May 1924 under the chairmanship of Sir John Anderson, who was the Permanent Under Secretary of State at the Home Office.

The entire matter of an ARP service was, from the outset, regarded as somewhat complex not only in its very wide remit, but also in the amount of co-operation needed from the many and varied government and external organisations in order to ensure compliance and implementation. For this reason it was considered essential to structure the committee with a cross-section of representatives from both military and civilian bodies, all of whom would be charged with making air raid precautions an effective part of home defence in a future war. In addition to the chairman, the committee comprised six members who represented the Committee of Imperial Defence, the Ministry of Health, the Office of Works and the Army, Royal Air Force and Royal Navy. Almost immediately the committee invited other members representing the General Post Office and the Board of Trade to join. From time to time, and as demands of the meetings required, invitations were extended to other organisations, including the Chemical Warfare Research Department.

The single most important task of this committee was to investigate and implement ways in which the civil authorities could come together to ensure that the activities of the fighting services were effective. With this term of reference, the chairman placed before the committee seven key subjects for discussion and examination. These subjects were legislative powers, departmental responsibility, the maintenance of vital services, how and when warnings would be given, prevention of damage, repair of damage and operation of the government. At a meeting shortly after the inaugural meeting, another main subject was added to this list. The education of the public in the significance of air attack was a matter which it was agreed should be discussed confidentially with 'reliable' people outside government circles. This subject of all of them was regarded as the most sensitive, in that information about air raids and the likely outcome of raids could cause panic if its presentation to the population was not delivered correctly. Within the first year of the committee's existence, the general managers of the country's four main railway companies were involved in talks which became necessary within the developing depth and width of the planning strategy.

Meanwhile, the Manpower Committee was giving consideration to a number of other matters. These were the perceived need for large numbers of men to engage in anti-aircraft duties and a preliminary investigation into the matter of early warnings and observation systems. Just as significant was the tremendous amount of examination undertaken on the dangers of air attacks, based on a series of anticipations and theories about the capabilities of modern aircraft and the lessons learned during the First World War. Interestingly, the conclusions were that in the first twenty-four hours of the outbreak of another war, an air attack on London would claim over 1,500 killed and over 3,000 wounded. In every subsequent period of twenty-four hours, a further 2,500 people would become casualties. These figures and arguments about the morale of the civilian population were presented to the ARP Committee, who were already facing a significant challenge as a result of all the other data that was being delivered to them through various internal and external representations. The problems of ARP were recognised in the committee's first report, which made meticulous proposals on each of the eight main subjects. Under each subject heading very many considerations were made and indications given as to the probabilities of need in terms of services, facilities and manpower. This information was based on the calculations of the Air Staff as to the frequency and severity of enemy attack from the air. Such likely attacks were regarded as being either 'mass attacks', which would cause widespread destruction and death, or lighter 'raids', which would be used by the enemy to panic and alarm the population.

Whereas mass attacks were considered reason to issue warnings to civil organisations, mere 'raids' apparently did not justify any form of advance notice. The warnings for imminent mass attacks were defined in two categories, with the first warning issued only to bodies such as the fire services, the police and organisations who needed time to put their anti-aircraft systems into operation. A second warning was to be given about fifteen or twenty minutes later when an attack was imminent. This would be timed to ensure minimum disruption of 'normal activities' as people went about their daily business.

'The men, women and children, the very citadel and heart of the nation's strength, were the care of the wardens and Rescue Workers', said a government statement of about 1940.

So what of the services on the ground during and after air raids? These services, such as ambulances and fire brigades, were recognised as needing additional manpower because resources were stretched during heavy attacks. With this in mind, the list sent to the Manpower Commission concerning the manning of anti-aircraft facilities also included allowances for the effective provision of emergency services. No real thought was given however, to the specialised needs of the ARP in fulfilling its duties, including gas decontamination.

In the following years, and during an increasing number of meetings at which numerous government and civilian organisations discussed, reviewed and endeavoured to move forward on an increasing agenda of strategic matters, various documents and papers were given consideration. These included 'The Supply of London in the event of the Port of London being wholly or partially closed', 'The Organisation of Medical

Services', 'The Protection of the Civil Population against Gas Attack' and, interestingly, a paper resulting from a study by the French government called 'Practical Instruction on Passive Defence against Air Attack'.

In 1933, a more detailed report was presented by the then recently designated Air Raids Commandant under the title of 'Memorandum on the preparation of a scheme for the Passive Defence of London against aerial bombardment'. London, as well as being the seat of government, was regarded as the best template upon which to base all such theories and plans, because if they worked in London they could easily be transplanted to other major towns and cities. In this report the author identified fifteen categories of ARP operations which would need to recruit civilians from the available pool of manpower, notwithstanding the need to strengthen the ranks of all the armed services.

It was recognised that,

> in organising the whole civilian population to protect themselves they must be organised on a civilian basis in their civilian organisations of the categories named. The ARP service must create and maintain its own honourable status and prestige and not lean upon some other service. It would be contrary to the principle of this civilian organisation to resist attack upon civilians if it were to be incorporated in the Territorial Army or any other military organisation.

Within the subsequent programme were details of the matters which were deemed as requiring immediate action, and also funding from the 1934–35 financial year budget. In addition to,

for example, the organisation of a full-scale air raid precaution exercise and a thorough test of the destructive capabilities of a 500 lb bomb, emphasis was also placed on the need to create a firefighting organisation on a huge scale that had never previously been envisaged, as well as the consolidation of the fire brigades operating in and serving London.

The implications of the cost of these projects was then considered, and the committee decided that they could not recommend any of them if the cost was 'prohibitive'. At the time, expenditure on passive defence was about £20,000 per year, much of which, incidentally, was being used by the Chemical Defence Department. The monies now being asked for by Major-General Pritchard, newly appointed Air Raids Commandant, were in the order of £150,000 over the following financial year, and it was decided that this could only be justified if the country was under serious threat of a maximum attack. The committee therefore chose to seek fresh guidance from the government as to what scale, this inevitably being guesswork of course, they should use to assist them in planning. The conclusion was that preparations could proceed temporarily without the need to rely on any references as to the scale of likely attacks, although it was acknowledged that attacks would be on a far greater scale than those experienced during the First World War. Effort was to be directed primarily towards organisation and material preparation, providing that no 'heavy' expenditure was involved. This plan of action was agreed in late 1933.

Despite the fact that air raids and the likely consequences for the British population in another war were matters which had been on the agenda and discussed since the last days of the previous war, and despite the government's acceptance of the need for air raid precautions, the whole business of implementing civil defence for the United Kingdom during the war years of 1939–45 began with much indifference and a belief that war could be avoided, at least as far as this nation was concerned. It was not so much a case of apathy; rather it was simply that the politicians and the population were unable to accept the reality of another war. Many still clung on to the belief that the First World War had been 'the war to end all wars', and it was only as a result of international events in 1938 did the realisation begin to strike.

So, when rather belatedly recognition was given to the fact that war would come, and it was only a matter of when rather than if, preparations for civil defence and its initial implementation were hit and miss. Recruitment of wardens fell far short of target, and the training of personnel was lax – as indeed was the provision of vital equipment.

William Cox remembers,

My father was something to do with the War Office, we never did know what, but my mother recalls him saying that the country had been steadily preparing for the inevitable since the mid-1930s and by 1938 when Chamberlain had temporarily appeased Adolf Hitler at the famous Munich meeting, instructions were given to all the government departments to go on a war footing and prepare for the worst. My mum volunteered for the WVS and she also later on led a firefighting party in our road.

Betty Hockey noted in her diary: 'Many say Prime Minister Chamberlain was blamed wrongly for meeting Hitler, but in the opinion of many others, the country was given a year to prepare and a stay of execution until that fateful day in September 1939 when Britain declared war on Germany.'

The Ministry of Home Defence, a new section within the Department of State, was established to administer, with local and central authorities and other 'institutions', the problems that the implementation of civil defence gave rise to. It is reasonable to say that administration, through a network of different organisations, was in itself responsible for many of the early problems and some of the ongoing problems associated with the deployment of men and women within the many 'sections' of civil defence. However, despite the problems associated with the need for effective communication, for example, and short supplies of equipment in one area with more than ample supplies in other sector areas, civil defence was beginning to prove itself as a vital and efficient organisation as it struggled to cope not only with the after-effects of air raids, but with manpower shortages, dealing with new forms of attack and maintaining and supplying special equipment.

For millions of ordinary citizens, other than those in the Armed Services, involvement with civil defence was inevitable. Either as a volunteer or as a victim of air raids, men, women and children depended on the activities of the first aid parties, the rescue crews or the wardens. Because the air offensive was an integral part of the enemy's strategy to force Britain to surrender, the balance between victory and defeat during certain stages of the war hung heavily in the balance. While destruction of property created a significant threat, it was the possibility of the 'destruction' of the population that caused the most alarm. Civil defence therefore, had to remain alert and staffed at all times, and throughout their years of service, the duties were to far exceed the immediate responsibility of helping to counter and deal with the impact of air attacks upon the population.

Notwithstanding these duties, the Civil Defence Service was one of several that had responsibility for defending Britain against air attack. The pre-eminent role of the Royal Air Force as a front-line defence was supported by the Observer Corps (later the Royal Observer Corps). Under the control of Fighter Command, the Corps was the prime source of intelligence for the entire defence structure with responsibility for monitoring and reporting upon the movement of hostile aircraft. Of equal importance was the Anti-Aircraft Command, upon whose shoulders fell the responsibility of shooting down as many enemy aircraft as possible before bombs and strafing could be unleashed upon the masses. The services were effectively divided into two categories, those of active and passive defences. With manpower and resources stretched to the limit, there was much debate at regional and national level as to where the resources should be directed. Passive defence of the nation was ultimately given more support, relative to other defence methods, than it had previously been given during the aerial bombardment of the country during the First World War.

Taken against the wider factor of the nation's (lack of) appetite for and (negative) attitude towards war (it was considered that the population was 'exhausted' and the slow process of financial recovery had had a negative impact on the lives of everyone), the first committee to examine the situation with regard to future attacks by enemy aircraft reported to government in 1922. During the twenty years of peace after the end of the First World War, the authorities therefore engaged in learning from the experiences of aerial bombardment and addressing the hypothetical threats against the country in another war. They concluded that 'the moral effect of air attack is out of all proportion to the material effect which it can achieve'. It was recognised, therefore, that the problem of the morale of the population in another war would be a crucial factor.

The temperament of the British, so it was judged, only became hostile when war was actually declared, and most people were reluctant to entertain the idea that another world war was probable. The lack of support for the planning of air raid precautions in the years before the outbreak of the Second World War was therefore understandable.

One commentator, James King, observed,

The British have never quite succeeded in taking a realistic view of the prospects before them. Many were paying lip service to the reality whilst taking the precautions advised by the government, making the necessary sacrifices and working like beavers to prepare. They dug trenches, learnt passwords, divided up limited stocks of ammunition, selected sites for mass graves and built shelters. They listened to discouraging reports of German tactics and cleared land for defensive purposes. When they felt they could give a good account of themselves, seemingly they still found it impossible to appreciate the terrible dangers which invasion was expected to throw at them.

3
A MEASURE OF NATIONAL IMPORTANCE

During the 1930s, the British government was reasonably well informed of activities in Germany which indicated that the country might be preparing for war.

It was reported through the 'usual sources', such as reports by visitors to the country and commercial awareness of industrial activities, as well as observations by the Intelligence Services, that there was an increase in the numbers of civilian flying schools, an expansion of the national Labour Corps and a widespread introduction of physical training for the population. Other indications too, including preparations to defend the country against aerial bombardment, led some politicians to believe that a real threat existed.

Britain was then alerted to the devastation caused by the techniques and 'success' of air raids against a civilian population and the subsequent fires which had disrupted Spain during the civil war which raged in that country during the late 1930s. This information came from the usual news sources as well as from British civilians who had volunteered to fight. A number of these civilians were to form what amounted to an unofficial advisory board upon their return to England. Meanwhile,

Britain's peacetime fire service was fragmented. A mix of local brigades and those serving factories and private estates, they were not trained or equipped at the time to cope with major emergencies. As previously noted, in some areas of the country including Manchester and Portsmouth, the police service was responsible for the provision of fire cover.

Ken Hampton, a retired Portsmouth police officer, remembers,

In my day there was no cadet or probationer service as there has been since the war. Back then you had the opportunity of either becoming an apprentice fireman in the city Police Force or a shorthand typist in the Criminal Investigation Bureau. This meant that you were basically a civilian but you were working under the auspices of the force. At the end of our service as apprentice firemen we would be sworn in as a constable and that was at age twenty. There was no question of us going away to training college, instead we went into local police classes for about ten or twelve weeks and we learnt police law and we did physical training. Incidentally we also learned firefighting as well. We were expected to take on most of the duties with the possible exception of running the pumps on the fire engine, which we were never asked to do.

Apart from lectures we had fire drills in the yard of one of the fire stations and then we were taught how to roll out lines of hoses, how to deal with chimney fires and also how to deal with major conflagrations. The other thing we had to do was sheet jumps from the tower, hoping that the sheet was held firmly when we landed in it.

Several other forces in the country also operated their local brigades but in Portsmouth we were unique because we ran the ambulance service as well. We used to drive the ambulances with qualified St John's personnel, although we too had to qualify in first aid as well as gaining a life-saving certificate. If you failed to get both these certificates, your services were dispensed with immediately.

With the introduction of the Air Raid Precautions Act (1937) and the Fire Brigades Act (1938), the attention of the British nation became focused on the need for planning and preparing for conflict, whenever it might come. The building of air raid shelters was a vital activity, parallel only to the urgent galvanisation and expansion of the country's 1,400 peacetime fire brigades. Almost overnight in 1937, it became the challenge of the Fire Brigades Division to organise the fire brigades of England and Wales and adapt them to the needs of a wartime role. Thus in those difficult times in Europe and worldwide, when war clouds loomed and the battle facing democracy was never greater, the Auxiliary Fire Service (AFS) was born. The AFS, all citizen volunteers, was to be a self-contained organisation which would work with the regular service to help meet and defeat the fires caused by air raids.

The official presentation of the need for the service stated that 'The Government has deemed it necessary to augment the existing Fire Brigade Service as a measure of national importance.'

The reasons for the creation of the service were many and varied, but there were five prime reasons. The nation's fire service would have to be organised to deal with the large number of fires which would be caused simultaneously by the dropping of incendiary bombs by enemy aircraft. The resulting damage could interfere with the supply of mains water supplies which the services would rely upon for firefighting, and so large numbers of men would need to be trained for the purpose of obtaining water supplies by trailer pump from more distant sources. In addition to pump duties, members of the service would also have to be available to maintain effective communication between stations and the general public in the event that the usual lines of communication were adversely affected by bomb damage.

During air raids it would be necessary to have all commercial and private property under supervision, and therefore fire crews would need to be of sufficient numbers to patrol the streets with mobile appliances to ensure that outbreaks were tackled immediately. Last but not least, heavy-duty mobile apparatus would need to be maintained at stations throughout the boroughs, in readiness to respond not only to major emergencies in the area, but also for duties in other areas and other parts of the country if needed.

Recruitment teams toured towns and cities as part of the campaign to attract applicants to the fire service. Every public house, post office and factory was a source of recruitment, while magazines and newspapers wrote again and again about the need for men and women to join the Fire Service. In the provinces however, training and equipment did, with few exceptions, fall some way behind the cities.

The resources of the regular fire brigades, although much improved by rafts of new legislation, were to be overshadowed by the expanding AFS. Fire risks in wartime presented a problem of such alarming proportions that a peacetime conception of adequate protection was not in the same realm of discussion as emergency planning. The government deemed it necessary to augment the existing fire brigade services as a measure of national importance. Calculations by the Home Office suggested that in an air attack by a single bomber over a closely populated area about seventy-five fires could break out over a distance of three miles along the flight path of the aircraft. A built-up area might experience some 150 fires alone, and a flight of ten bombers would increase these numbers pro rata. Purely on a cost and manpower basis it was soon realised that it would be impossible to provide fire cover for all areas at all times. Instead, the intention was to ensure that every major community settlement of more than 20,000 inhabitants and major areas including industrial centres and railway junctions had an emergency organisation capable of dealing with fairly intensive bombing.

The AFS then expanded substantially, and as a consequence it demanded men, machines and equipment in huge numbers. Although members of the regular fire service, that is the service which had provided peacetime cover, had benefited from the availability of more resources, organisationally they were not immediately regarded as being up to the challenges of a wartime or extreme emergency situation. Even with the regular firemen being given exemption from war service as a result of their roles being classified as reserved occupations, this in itself did not allay the overall problems of bringing the fire service up to wartime strength through the recruitment and training of enough men and women to supplement the regulars.

Previously, in 1936, an arrangement had been made whereby regular firemen who had also enlisted as reservists in the Armed Services would not be called up immediately upon the declaration of war. This took into account the fact that a number of professional fire brigades, including the London Fire Brigade, had traditionally recruited naval reservists.

Recruitment for volunteers to join the AFS began in earnest in early 1937, when those not in the Armed Services and between the ages of twenty-five and fifty years were encouraged to volunteer. Apart from lectures and 'exercises', including the burning of slum dwellings, the authorities promoted the recruitment drive through a poster campaign and newspaper features, with photographs showing men and women lying flat on their stomachs putting out incendiary bombs with stirrup pumps. The stirrup pump was in fact an adapted piece of equipment from the nineteenth century. Later, canteen vans were fitted with loudspeakers for the purpose of taking the message to the heart of the community, and it wasn't long before towns and cities in many parts of England were following this lead.

Once recruited, volunteers had to undergo a recommended sixty-hour training programme based on a syllabus set out in the memo of February 1937. The memo also emphasised the need for refresher courses to be implemented at regular intervals and, whenever possible, auxiliaries were to be given the opportunity to gain practical experience in firefighting in 'peace time'.

Steve Long said his grandfather volunteered for service,

He said his crew were taken to a quarry somewhere and it was full of water. They had to practise drawing the water from the site and using it to put out a fire that had been lit in a nearby abandoned hut. Unfortunately they did not have all the right equipment on the appliance and the hut was left to burn itself out.

Standard training meanwhile addressed challenges that included the handling and use of appliances (later called trailer pumps), entering a burning building to test personal endurance in intense heat and dense smoke and carrying a disorientated person down a ladder.

Initially, the training of new recruits fell to the members of the regular fire service; however, as auxiliaries became competent in the required skills, many were, in turn, able to train new recruits. The matter of training, though, raised challenges of a different kind. A shortage of suitable premises resulted in many training sessions being conducted in a number of makeshift venues, including garages and shops. Improvisation was the order of the day, as it was across most of the Civil Defence Service. And when the number of new recruits increased, the recommended sixty hours of training had to be condensed into a shortened version. As venues became full of trainees, it was a Herculean task to provide the full sixty-hour programme, because resources were stretched to the limit.

The eighty-two-page AFS General Training Manual gave all the basic information a new recruit would need from how to find your way out of a building ('the easiest method of finding a way out of a smoke filled building is to follow the hose back to the point of entry') to dealing with unexploded bombs ('notify the responsible authority as laid down in instructions and until their arrival keep all persons well clear').

The original memo of February 1937 also gave advice on the provision of uniforms and equipment for auxiliaries, although it was for the individual authorities to adopt a type and style of uniform that they felt best served the purpose. However, in 1938, recruits were to be issued with 'authorised uniforms and equipment' as per a standard design and style consisting of overalls, cap, boots, belt and axe while in training and tunic, trousers and oilskin leggings when required for 'wet' drills. Sometime in 1939 a waterproof coat was issued. Female members of the AFS were also provided with a standard uniform designed to meet the needs of the work upon which they were engaged. Cap badges, breast badges and buttons were produced by the Post Office Stores Department and sent out to all the authorities. A buttonhole badge was issued for the use of AFS members when off duty.

Cyril Kendall was an experienced fireman based in Reading, Berkshire,

In 1938 a lot of the fire brigades amalgamated and our brigade took on a number of newly recruited Auxiliary Fire Service men. Our job was to prepare the vehicles and the men themselves and because I had previously had a commission in the Army Cadet Force it was easy for me to organise everything in a practical manner along military lines. For a year or so I gave training in pump drill and ladder drill and it was a very interesting time.

Training also covered drills associated with drawing water from rivers and water tanks as well as from hydrants. Additionally the training included 'How to Act in Various Emergencies', everything from the fire appliances being 'rendered useless' to how to deal with broken water mains.

By late 1938, considerable progress had been made. Training establishments now neared some 2,500 in number and 13,000 auxiliaries had successfully completed the standard course. Of the 82,000 people enrolled, over 50,000 were still in training, and some local authorities had carried out exercises to familiarise pump crews and control room staff with operational procedures.

While the basic principle of civil defence work was that it was of an unpaid voluntary nature, it was obvious to government that conditions of service and pay would have to be addressed and agreed for those volunteers who in an emergency would become full-time workers. This was especially true of the AFS for, as the Home Office realised, this service would require a larger number of full-time members than would the other civil defence services. The recognised and special characteristic of efficient firefighting is speed, and to achieve this especially in areas considered as being 'high risk' it would be vital to have the necessary contingents of full-timers. It was important therefore, that details of the pay and conditions for the men and women who volunteered for possible full-time service should be made available in good time, so that those who might serve in this capacity would know what to expect.

The government made an announcement in February 1939 when it had reached the decision to pay a weekly amount of £3 to the male and £2 to the female volunteers. Attention now focused on another matter that had been given thought and consideration over many months: the government needed to assess with some accuracy the numbers of AFS personnel who would be available for full-time duty in an emergency. The following month, March, saw the publication of figures sourced from the local fire authorities, which indicated their estimate of numbers of personnel that were going to be needed to effectively cope with an emergency. The figure quoted was 175,000, although this was in stark contrast to the estimate of nearly 300,000 that the Home Office had predicted.

In the event of hostilities, it was recognised that members of the AFS would be confronted with a diverse range of emergencies, and although there were guidelines as to how to deal with them, it was acknowledged that a great deal would depend on the prevailing circumstances and the self-reliance and 'promptitude' of individual AFS members.

A decision about the purchase and supply of major equipment had already been made, and such items were to be purchased centrally and loaned out to the various authorities with priority given to authorities in high-risk areas. The main reason for this decision was that no manufacturing capability existed at the time for the production of appliances and equipment in the quantities needed.

The large and differing collection of fire authorities had in the past bought their engines and other equipment in small numbers, perhaps only a single item at a time. To make the investment in plant and machinery, manufacturers needed to take orders in greater numbers in order to successfully achieve speed and capacity of production. This was especially so with regard to the production of pumps, which from the beginning were recognised as the most important and most urgently needed piece of equipment. Pumps on their own, of course, were useless, and a list of over 120 different ancillary items of equipment had to be fulfilled within the vast manufacturing process. These items included 100,000 nozzles, 45,000 medium-sized ladders up to a length of 30 feet and 50,000 branch pipes. In addition, large numbers of motor vehicles were required for towing trailer pumps, hose laying, for carrying water and for use as platforms for turntable ladders.

The Office of Works was realistically the only department able to organise and manage the production and buying in of equipment on such a scale. They were familiar too with the likely engineering challenges that may arise. So it came about that as soon as technical specifications, drawings and delivery schedules had been arranged between the Home Office and the Office of Works, contracts were immediately placed with suitable suppliers, including Sulzer and Dennis Bros of Guildford, Surrey, who began the manufacture of heavy pumps to the prescribed standard design.

However, a situation which had not previously been considered by those responsible for planning and executing the terms of reference for the fire service had arisen, and needed urgent resolution. Under what circumstances were emergency appliances to be lent to local authorities? The ARP provided powers to the Secretary of State to acquire equipment 'for the purpose of affording protection to persons and property from injury or damage in the event of hostile attack from the air' and further 'to make loans, gifts or sales of such equipment'. That said, the Act did not allow for the use of appliances other than in an emergency and so, as it stood, auxiliary firemen would be deprived of the use of suitable

equipment for much needed training in their peacetime role. To overcome this hurdle, a new clause known as Section 21 was inserted into the Fire Brigades Act, providing for a more flexible supply and use of equipment. But the Treasury were anxious to ensure that fire authorities should not become reliant on loaned equipment, manned by auxiliaries to fill any shortfalls in the delivery of their existing peacetime services, thereby effectively evading their responsibilities of the Fire Brigades Act. By the end of 1938, new rules were in place, and these specifically laid down the conditions under which equipment could be supplied on loan.

The appliances might be used in peace time for maintenance purposes, for training and for extinguishing fires in exceptional circumstances when necessary to save life and property, and when local equipment was insufficient or not readily available. The local authority had to keep the appliances in good working order and might be held responsible for repairing any damage or replacing any loss (the cost would be reimbursed if the peacetime fire was being used as a training fire), it must keep records of the use of the equipment and allow it to be inspected as required.

No one could be in any doubt that the task ahead, that of a large-scale and quite rapid expansion, was substantial, and the likely complications would be many and varied. However, a key decision was taken that the manufacturing effort should be on trailer pumps of various categories, heavy, large, medium and light. Painted in battleship grey, these pumps, with the exception of the heavy variety, were to become a familiar sight on the streets as they were towed to incidents behind lorries and cars. Initially it was thought that local authorities could requisition the required numbers of suitable towing vehicles when war came, but this was not to be, and many authorities had to purchase second-hand high-powered cars and a small number of lorries. This arrangement too broke down, and it was necessary to purpose-build vehicles and loan them to local authorities.

Trailer pumps were manufactured on a national basis by eleven different companies, each of whom had a degree of flexibility when it came to incorporating their own ideas and special build features. While it is reasonable to think that a standard design pump would have been more time and cost effective, to incorporate the ideas and needs of all the brigades would have entailed considerable research and experiment. There was simply no time to engage in such activities. Nor was there much time to deliberate on the exact numbers of pumps that would be required, and so a number of calculations were made based on the information gleaned from the reports of aerial bombardment and the likely damage caused by incendiary bombs.

The first serious estimate, which also took into account the needs of local authorities in terms of the areas they served, was for between 17,000 and 21,000 units, added to which was ancillary equipment including 3,000 miles of hose. This estimate was quite accurate, in that the units were gradually phased in and reasonably met the needs of the fire services by the time of the heavy air raids during 1940 and 1941.

By about mid-year in 1938, orders had already been placed for ancillary equipment and for pumps at a total cost of £1,000,000, although delivery was slow and just a handful of pumps, some 420, had been delivered of the total 20,000 required

for operational service in a (the) coming war. At the time of the Munich Crisis, London had less than 100 pumps, but had recruited over 13,000 AFS personnel. Herbert Morrison, who was at the time the Leader of London County Council, said, 'It is shameful, that these volunteers who have come forward to do a very dangerous job should be short of the essential appliances.' In fact, at the time that this criticism was made, the order for pumps had already been increased from 4,500 to nearly 7,000.

In November 1938, the target date given for the completion of the production programme of all the pumps and equipment ordered was spring 1941, a date very much based on the assumptions made by the Air Ministry in 1937 as to the type, size and duration of an aerial attack on the country. Thankfully though, in December 1938 the various departments involved in the production programme took steps to accelerate the equipment deliveries and bring forward the completion date to early 1940. In early 1939, after a little deliberation by the Treasury, further orders were placed which bought the total up to 26,900 machines.

By May 1939, the chief officers of the various fire brigade areas were able to put forward a figure of 65,000 potential full-time firemen from the 140,000 AFS members by then recruited. It was interesting to note the fact that the work of the 4,500 women in the AFS was finally being recognised as making a positive impact, particularly in tasks such as driving, telephone operation and watch room control.

By June 1939, when nearly 900 'schemes' (local and rural district councils who became part of the coordinated programme for firefighting under the ARP Act) had been received and approved, the AFS had 120,000 men with 18,000 watch room attendants as well as a large number of women and young men engaged in various essential duties including despatch riders and cooks. Over 4,250 appliances were by then in service and in excess of 450 miles of new hose had been issued in addition to the supply of other equipment. In November of the same year, the Inspectorate of Fire Brigades, which had been initiated in March 1937, had appointed one inspector and one assistant to each of the Regional Commissioners Headquarters and a chief inspector and two engineering inspectors were installed at the Home Office. As one commentator asked glibly, 'Who would dare set fire to London now?'

On 1 September 1939, the order for Action Stations was given by radio broadcast and by telephone to the men and women of the AFS. From many factories, offices, shops and farms, they rushed to their designated stations in preparation for the ensuing emergency. Two days later, on the outbreak of war, about 60 per cent of all equipment was actually in service with the brigades around the country, and the men and women were ready for whatever challenges lay ahead.

Winston Churchill, speaking in the House of Commons, said,

As I see it, we must so arrange that, when any district is smitten by bombs, which are flung about at utter random, strong mobile forces will descend on the scene in power and mercy to conquer the flames. We have to make a job of this business of living and working under fire.

Long dark months of trials and tribulations lie before us. Death and sorrow will be the companions of our journey, constancy and valour our only shield. We must be united, we must be undaunted. Our qualities and deeds must burn and glow through the gloom of Europe until they become the veritable beacon of its salvation.

At the time of Churchill's speech and before September 1940, 80 per cent of London's auxiliary firemen had never fought a fire.

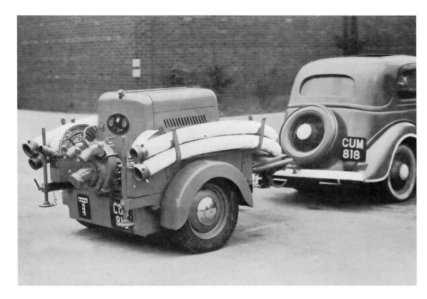

Left: A trailer pump towed behind a private car in this early war image.

Right: A typical blitz scene witnessed by members of the CCFF, although the exact location is unclear.

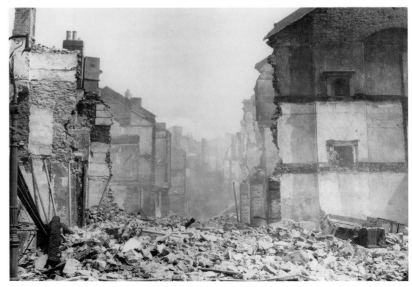

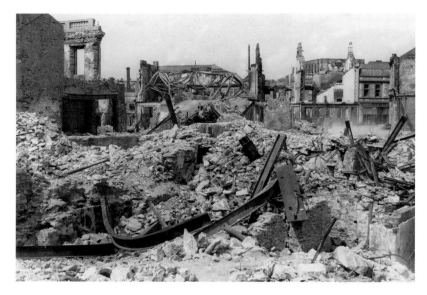

Right: More devastation of the type dealt with by contingents of the CCFF with their NFS colleagues.

Left: Another street scene after a raid as experienced by the men of the Corps.

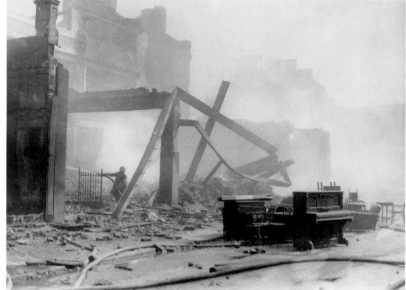

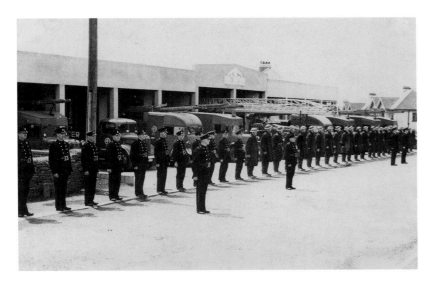

The Plymouth
Right: One of the mess huts used by the corps from 1942.

New Appliances
Left: New appliances which were issued to the Corps in Plymouth, 1942.

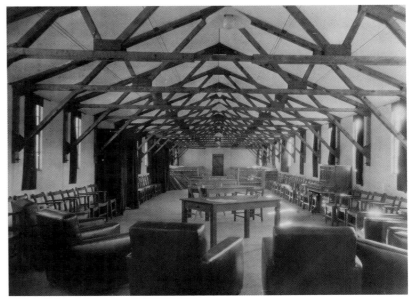

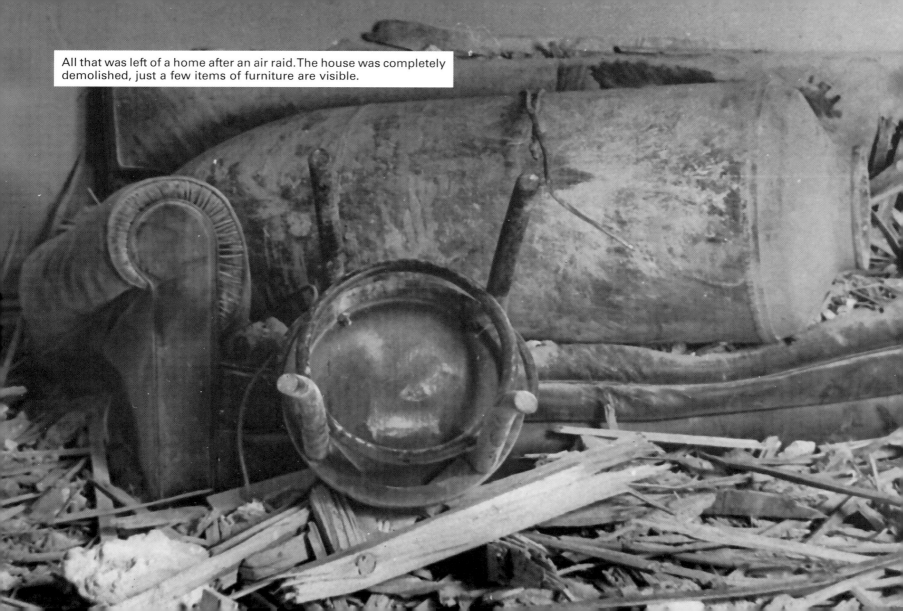

All that was left of a home after an air raid. The house was completely demolished, just a few items of furniture are visible.

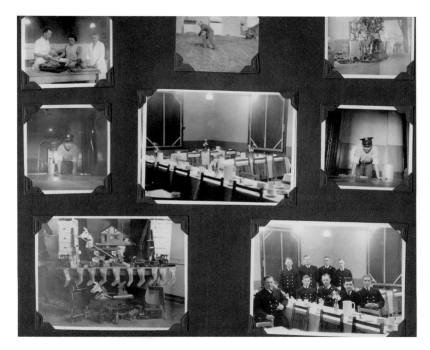

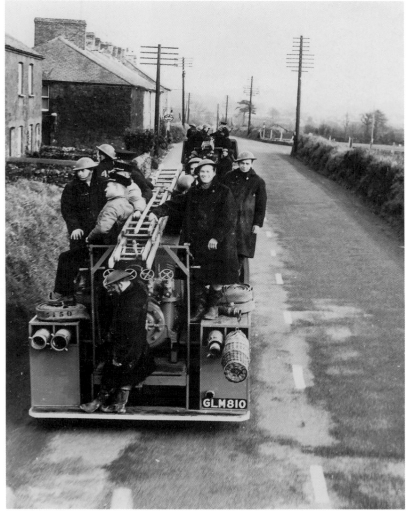

Aftermath of a Blitz Raid
Above: Personal photographs showing Corps members preparing for Christmas.

Right: Corps members on duty crewing an NFS fire appliance.

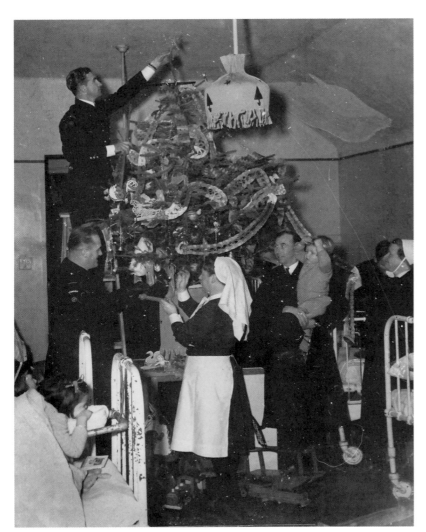

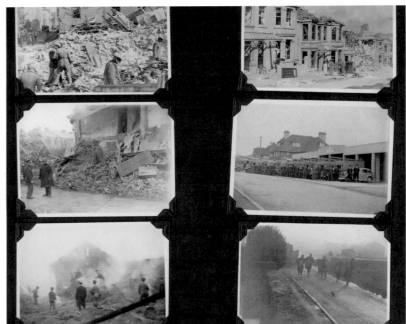

Christmas 1942
Above: More personal photographs showing Blitz damage and the station at Plymouth.

A CCF Crew
Left: Corps members visit a local hospital to bring a little cheer to the children.

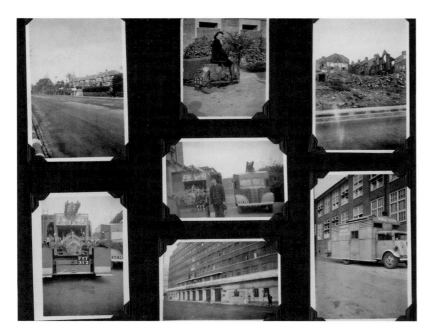

Above and right: Personal Photos

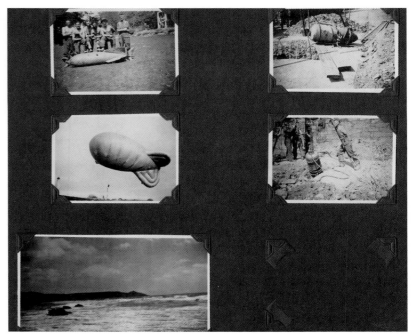

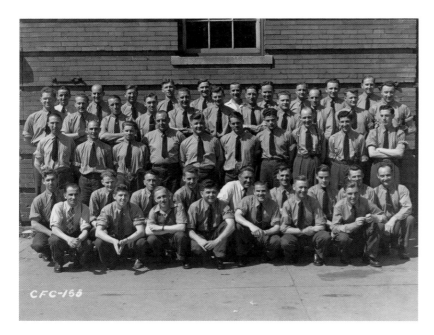

Canadians in Southampton
Above: The Southampton contingent of the Corps, who were billeted near the docks at the Apollo Hotel.

Left: Personal Photos

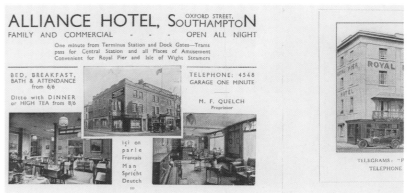

ALLIANCE HOTEL, SOUTHAMPTON OXFORD STREET,
FAMILY AND COMMERCIAL - - - OPEN ALL NIGHT

One minute from Terminus Station and Dock Gates—Trams
pass for Central Station and all Places of Amusement
Convenient for Royal Pier and Isle of Wight Steamers

BED, BREAKFAST,
BATH & ATTENDANCE
from 6/6

Ditto with DINNER
or HIGH TEA from 8/6

TELEPHONE: 4548
GARAGE ONE MINUTE

M. F. QUELCH
Proprietor

ici on
parle
Francais
Man
Spricht
Deutch

ROYAL

TELEGRAMS: "P
TELEPHONE.

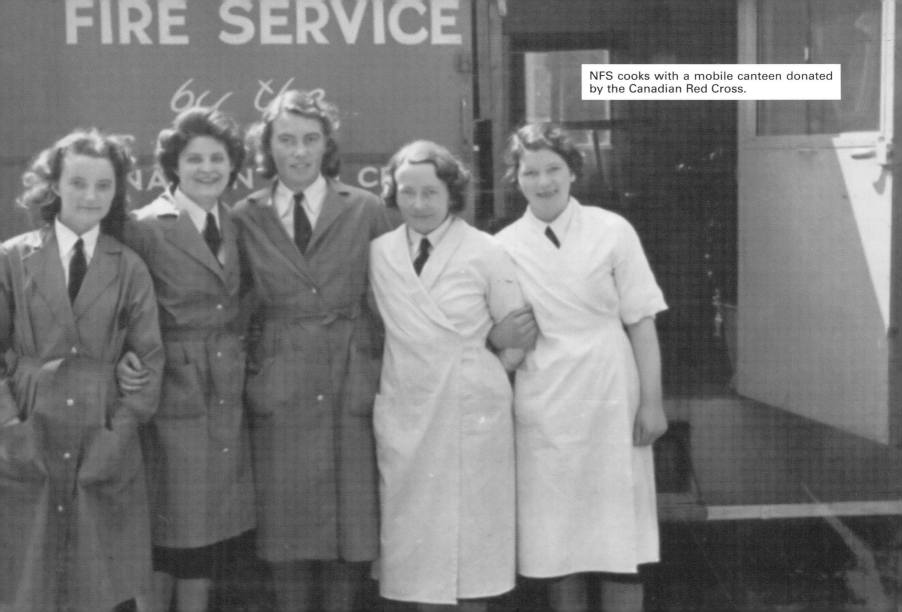

NFS cooks with a mobile canteen donated by the Canadian Red Cross.

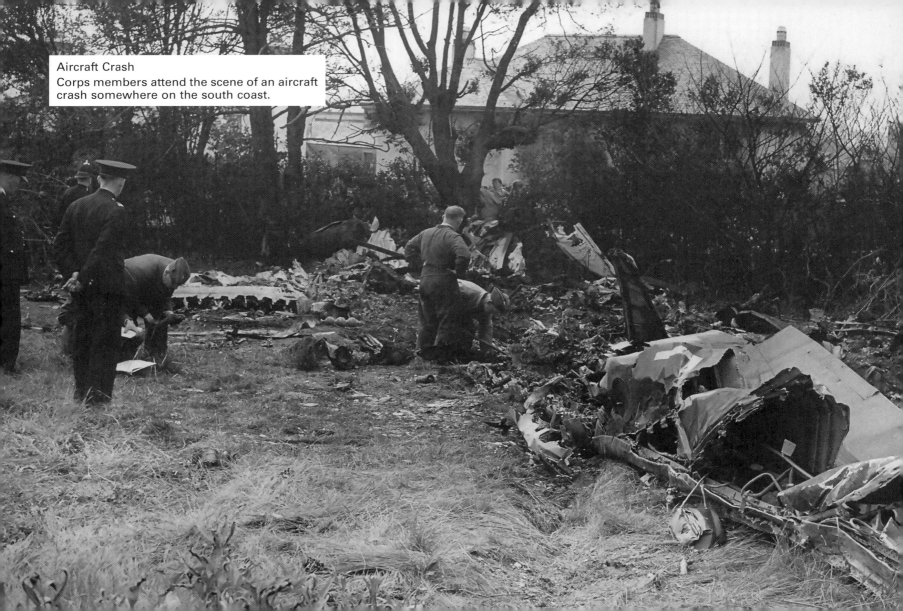

Aircraft Crash
Corps members attend the scene of an aircraft crash somewhere on the south coast.

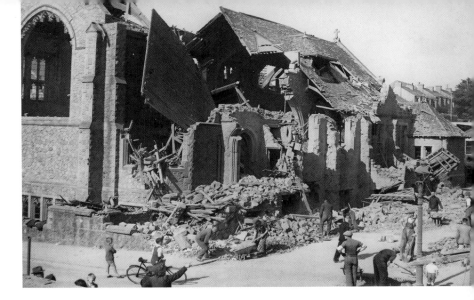

Plymouth
Above and below: Typical scenes in the blitzed city of Plymouth.

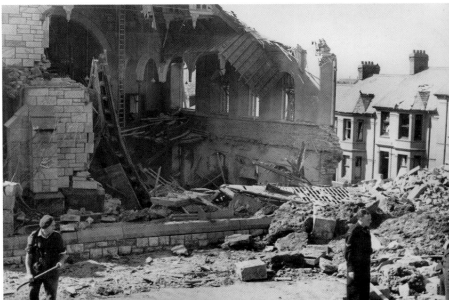

4

ACTIVE DEFENCES

The AFS, the Regular Fire Service and all the volunteer works brigades and stirrup pump parties were called to their posts just before the official declaration of war in September 1939, in full readiness for what lay ahead.

The whole matter of the possible consequences of air raids and of widespread destruction had been discussed and considered for many years and as long ago as the last years of the First World War. After various reports from 'think tanks', from the military and from those charged with planning civil defence, the matter of new measures to ensure effective firefighting in wartime conditions on the Home Front was to be placed firmly on the agenda. Some progress had been made as far as developing the 'shape' of emergency firefighting during 1937, and in this particular year it could be sensed that talking was now giving way to action and positive moves as far as the provision of fire cover in wartime was concerned.

The existing fire service consisted of 1,400 individual brigades and authorities and was, by its very nature, fragmented and without any cohesion or structure. Moreover, local authorities were under no obligation to provide peacetime fire cover, and the legislation was confusing and inadequate and resulted in many areas of the country having little or no fire service provision. Some brigades were well equipped, others had just a single-hand pump appliance, and very little appeared to have changed from the embryonic years of the fire service as it dragged itself into the twentieth century. Hose couplings and hosepipes varied from place to place and the service from one town, for example, could not assist in emergency firefighting in another because hoses did not fit the pumps. Communications between fire services in neighbouring towns and cities was almost non-existent. For the most part, the complement of men and machines was in no way commensurate with the needs of the expanding conurbations served, although the London Fire Brigade was, as an exception, both of a size and efficiency to provide for the demands made upon it in peacetime.

In 1935, attention had been drawn to the need for a coordinated fire service on a large scale to deal with major conflagrations and emergencies in which perhaps hundreds of people were involved. In writing one memorandum, the Home Officer Fire Adviser (HOFA) for London made mention of the fact that in another war the menace of the newly developed light incendiary device and the increasing range and capacity of aircraft would significantly increase the likelihood of widespread damage by fire. However, in what was known as the First Circular on air raid precautions, published in July of that year, hardly any mention was made of firefighting. The publication of this circular, though, was to virtually coincide with the creation of another new committee, the Riverdale Committee, which had the responsibility of looking at the matter of the existing fire service and of fulfilling the requirements to somehow mobilise it into an effective and cohesive national organisation.

There was beginning to emerge now, in some quarters, a greater recognition of the situations that might face a wartime fire service particularly if incendiaries were dropped over built-up and densely populated or industrialised areas of the country. Although a scheme of what was known as 'mutual re-enforcement' had been trialled in the First World War, this in itself would not be sufficient to address firefighting and the challenges of air raids in another war. The fire service would need to be considerably expanded, and it was further recognised that additional support would be needed from both the ARP services and the public in dealing with various types of localised and major fires.

Events elsewhere in the world were to bring home the realisation of the potential devastation that could be inflicted on Britain by aerial bombardment, and harsh lessons would be learnt if the country failed to grasp the significance of those events in Spain. From the outbreak of the Spanish civil war in July 1936, the Germans and the Italians had intervened and had taken every opportunity to practise and understand the techniques and success of bombing 'live' targets. Practising 'modern' warfare in this scenario undoubtedly assisted the Germans in applying and fine-tuning their military skills.

It is difficult to assess how much of the intelligence gathered in Spain was taken into consideration by the authorities at the time, given that there is no evidence of major changes in government thinking or policy. At the very least, though, the intelligence did serve to reinforce the fact that air raids on Britain were a viable and purposeful option for an enemy.

A detailed memo, the Emergency Fire Brigade Organisation, was issued by the Home Office in 1937, and this document might be generally regarded as the basis upon which the measures for wartime firefighting were founded.

Each of the brigades and authorities were asked to consider the matter of emergency firefighting and to devise plans to deal with such emergencies in their areas. To assist them in devising such plans, the Home Office memo gave terms of reference, and these included a number of headings not necessarily in order of importance. These were the 'Organisation of auxiliary fire stations', 'Augmentation of heavy appliances', 'Fire patrols and light trailer pumps', 'Vehicles for towing trailer pumps', 'Recruitment and Training of reserves and auxiliary firemen', 'Water Supplies including static supplies' and, last but not least, 'Emergency communications'. In recognition of the perceived need for the production and distribution of substantial quantities of equipment, hoses and appliances, a central purchasing and supply organisation would have to be set up, and this matter, as with those of finance and recruitment, were explained in guidelines provided with the memo. In essence, the cost of the expansion of the fire service to the levels anticipated for emergency duties would be funded through government loans and grants to the authorities, although such funding was taken in the wider context of the cost of providing ARP services as well. Some financing arrangements were to change, however, when the ARP Act of December 1937 provided for the loan of many items of emergency equipment.

The recruitment of volunteers for the AFS (fit and able volunteers with no firefighting experience who were willing to serve in an emergency) began in earnest in early 1937 with simple criteria. Volunteers were to be between the ages of twenty-five and fifty years, be able to pass a medical examination and be prepared to be on duty in an emergency. It was recognised that training was paramount, if for no other immediate reason that to keep the new recruits 'interested', and with this in mind a training schedule was worked out for local implementation by each fire authority. The sixty-hour training programme was often delivered in a shortened format when authorities suddenly found themselves with an influx of volunteers and congestion at the training centre, as previously mentioned. Nevertheless, every volunteer had to learn the basic skills of handling pumps and appliances, rescues from a burning building and firefighting, with others learning how to operate a control centre.

What was being raised was the possibility of increasing the existing fire service provision across the country to up to ten times its existing strength, with such a service being a core component of the country's civil defence structure. Of course the proposal to expand the service was for the most part based on calculations, assumptions, studies and hypotheses which had been carried out by various bodies during the interwar years and which had some elements of 'worst case scenarios' built

in as a margin for safety. Local authorities were expected to address issues such as recruitment of men and organisation of auxiliary stations while adhering to the 'structure' and 'spirit' of the overall plan.

Helpfully, the Home Office had already devised a benchmark by which the likely needs of firefighting in different areas could be assessed. This benchmark comprised factors including the identification of street mileage and the geographical layout of the community, available manpower and local resources for water to include rivers and streams. They had also identified three types of fire risk, simply known as A, B and C. Large businesses, warehouses, department stores, factories, docks, timber yards, railway depots, oil storage depots and munitions stores were understandably regarded as a major risk under category A. Small shops and garages, yards, warehouses of no more than three storeys in height and similar constructions were regarded as category B and residential premises were in category C.

In March 1938, the Secretary of State introduced the Air Raid Precautions (Fire Schemes) Regulations, and these actually set out what each scheme was to embrace as well as introducing new factors, namely the 'securing' of suitable vehicles and the storage and maintenance of materials and equipment. Throughout England and Wales, empowerment was handed to rural district councils (RDCs) to submit suitable schemes for their areas, taking into consideration the main requirements of fire patrols and fire posts, the organisation of an emergency fire service and arrangements for the use of both natural and static supplies of water. The RDCs were not compelled to submit schemes, whereas urban authorities were under an obligation to prepare emergency ARP fire schemes, having of course been given an indication as to the likely scale of preparations needed and perhaps, more importantly at the time, the manner in which an expansion of the fire service would be financed. Meanwhile, the Secretary of State was given the power to organise special fire training centres and also to appoint fire brigade inspectors, who were charged with ensuring that the Act was being undertaken.

It was recognised that the task of completing the relevant forms in response to the government call was a major undertaking, and although there was something of an urgency about the process, the information that was to be submitted in the following months proved a valuable aid to gaining a more realistic overview of the state of the country's firefighting capabilities both in a peacetime role and as it prepared for an emergency situation. A scheme, once submitted by a local authority, had to be scrutinised and then assessed for the number of men, machines and fire stations likely to be approved under available grant funding. Each scheme would also be considered for the number of appliances which could be made available on loan; and already, in this regard, His Majesty's Office of Works was placing orders for the manufacture of such equipment.

In the spring of 1938, with approval being given for just 130 of the near 1,000 schemes expected, 360 emergency pumps had been supplied and some 30,000 firemen had been recruited. There were provisos attached to the approval of schemes in rural district areas, not least of which was the one set by the Treasury. They were sensitive to the fact that 'some districts' might overstate their needs so as to completely fund the provision of appliances, men and stations at the expense of the Treasury. In this respect, therefore, rural districts had to satisfy the relevant department that the peacetime fire cover was already in place and adequate, and further, no equipment was provided on loan until the 'vulnerability' of each area had been assessed.

The Fire Brigades Act was to receive Royal Assent on 28 July 1938 and the Act was based, for the most part, on the earlier recommendations of the Riverdale Committee. This Act stated that borough, urban and district councils, excluding London, were to 'be obliged' to provide or arrange for the establishment of an efficient fire brigade. The councils throughout England and Wales were to become 'fire brigade authorities', although parish councils were exempt from this legislation. Rural district councils were empowered to act for the parishes. The gaping hole in the process and the Achilles heel of the entire operation of expansion was that administration for the service still rested with the 1,440 separate fire brigades. Although at the time the nation's regular fire brigade had a strength of just over 6,500 men with another 13,000 as reservists, the act of administering any activity involving thousands of personnel across thousands of square miles was 'vulnerable'. This situation was not satisfactorily addressed until the formation of the NFS a few years later in 1941.

The needs of London were addressed in terms of a 'special mention', and although they applied for an emergency fire scheme just as other local authorities were doing, the situation in the capital was viewed differently. Interestingly, given the climate of the times, their original application for 2,500 trailer pumps and the recruitment of an additional 30,000 men was rejected; and it was not until January 1940 that approval was finally given for an establishment of 20,000 men and the provision of over 2,800 pumps.

In July 1939, organisations employing large numbers of people in all industrial centres were compulsorily made to provide blast- and splinter-proof shelters for their workers.

Balanced against the need to organise the defence organisations was the secrecy needed to avoid provocation of the enemy. Bringing civil defence to a state of readiness and carrying out evacuation, manning the air raid warnings and lighting arrangements could not have been done however, without widespread publicity. But there was a climate of urgency, and on 22 August 1939 the Cabinet took the first major step by calling up the active defences against air raids. These were the Royal Air Force fighter squadrons, the anti-aircraft guns and searchlight crews, the balloon barrage crews and those who operated the warning systems. Ministers were meeting on a daily basis, and from these meetings information was disseminated as necessary either for internal use or for wider circulation to the public. Local authorities were directed to act on certain aspects of the full local war instructions that had been issued several months previously, and the ARP Department began issuing a large number of circulars which helped to reinforce earlier instructions.

In collaboration with the newly formed Women's Voluntary Service, the government had made elaborate plans for the mass evacuation of an estimated four million people (mothers, children and invalids) from the 'danger zones'. At the outbreak of war, one and a half million Anderson shelters had been distributed to the poorest households, and there was provision for the distribution of about a million more free shelters.

At 11.15 a.m. on the morning of Sunday 3 September, two days after the firemen and women were called to Action Stations, the Prime Minister broadcast to the nation:

This morning the British Ambassador in Berlin handed the German government a final note stating that, unless we heard from them by 11 o'clock that they were prepared at once to withdraw their troops from Poland, a state of war would exist between us. I have to tell you now that no such undertaking has been received, and that consequently this country is at war with Germany.

The majority of the population had already, during the previous weeks, been occupied in preparations for war, and that final confirmation caused an understandable pause in the great pursuit of mobilisation and preparation. In Whitehall, ministers and officials who were engaged in the most urgent of matters gathered up their papers and gas masks and hurried to the basements below.

Now all the planning of the past years was to be implemented. The use of public shelters, the effectiveness of early warning systems, anti-aircraft, communications, fire prevention and extinction, the complete civil defence operation was now at war and as ready as they could be, knowing that the country was confronted by a threat more deadly than had previously been experienced.

The consensus of opinion in the government and the military was that the enemy would likely attack immediately in what was referred to as an 'all-out lightning air attack'. The fact that neither this threat, nor Churchill's warning that long dark months of trials and tribulations lay ahead, materialised from the outset should not divert attention away from the historical reality of the time. Within a matter of months, following the period of the Phoney War, the country was indeed under attack, and major cities including London were being 'blitzed' by the enemy. Further, the population remained on full alert for possible gas attacks, and training for this scenario continued to take place.

It was also during the months of the Phoney War that the men and women of the fire services continued to ready themselves for what was to come. The delivery of equipment including trailer pumps and appliances continued slowly towards achieving the 'numbers' proposed by the authorities in the immediate pre-war years. Where necessary, private cars and commercial vehicles were requisitioned and adapted for service to help maintain the mobility of fire crews. That said, there were a number of incidents across the country where brigades were short of vehicles, and an example in one dock area of a city of crews that had to push trailer pumps to incidents, highlighting the shortcomings in the grand plan of effective fire cover in time of war. One seaport refused to provide its fire officers with cars, with a leading alderman saying that he 'was not going to have officers gallivanting about the place in cars'. Clearly the reasons behind a mobile fire brigade had passed this man by.

Despite the respite afforded the country and the opportunities for the fire services to better prepare and equip, members of the AFS were accused by certain factions of being 'draft dodgers', because they were regarded as trying to avoid conscription into the fighting services. Those accusers were soon to eat their words when the enemy began their air attacks on major cities, for it was then that the fire services and the men and women of the AFS in particular faced challenges the like of which had never been seen or experienced in Britain. All aspects of the planning for, training in and implementation of firefighting in a wartime emergency were harnessed and put to the test.

Many of the early shortcomings had been dealt with by the time the heavy raids of 1940 were over, but that did not detract from the principal weaknesses in the system. A new assessment was required to ascertain whether the existing system was able to meet and defeat the demands which might continue to be made upon it. The menace of the light incendiary bomb and its effectiveness as an aerial weapon had now been established. The 1941 raids on London and Coventry proved beyond doubt that saturation incendiary bombing by the enemy was a successful strategy. The problem of fire and fire limitation particularly in large towns and cities remained the prime concern of the fire services and the various civil defence organisations. It was thought that the initial bombing campaign might lead to further much heavier raids with deadlier consequences. In that situation the fire services would be greatly handicapped by the weaknesses in the local brigade organisation. The possibility of an all-out attack on Britain was still likely, given the enemy's capabilities and strategy of aggression in mainland Europe, and from 1941 fire defence measures were therefore given a greater share of the resources for civil defence. More emphasis was placed on the planning of firefighting, and the subsequent and most important development was the nationalisation of the fire services, which was approved by the War Cabinet in May of that year. (Germany also nationalised its fire services during the war. Its services had previously been organised locally.)

Speaking on behalf of the government the Home Secretary Herbert Morrison said that to continue to meet the air attacks on the scale that had been experienced so far, 'a drastic change of organisation must be made'. He added: 'It is certainly my very definite view that after the war the firefighting forces should again be a local authority service.'

The organisational structure was overhauled to improve reporting and communication, new stations were built or acquired, additional supplies of hoses, piping, pumps and appliances were to be made available, training was revised and more recruits were called for. In the months following the change of fire provision to the NFS, the expected heavy incendiary raids did not come; instead the enemy engaged in what were called tip and run raids, most of which were on coastal areas. They caused little problem to the service and were of no great intensity, but in 1942 what were known as the Baedeker raids on cathedral cities proved to be the first great test for the NFS. Exeter, Bath, Canterbury and York were among the cities that suffered these reprisal raids.

The new NFS handbook included instructions for Out of District calls,

The NFS is now a mobile force unit which may be called from the safer areas to badly blitzed centres at a moment's notice. Such units may well be gone from their home stations for some days and while their food and rest are the responsibility of the Force they have gone to assist they must carry iron rations blankets etc in case the aided authority with the best of intentions is unable to cater adequately for them.

Each man would also be advised to carry shaving tackle, change of socks and shirt perhaps a reserve packet of cigarettes or tobacco and a little extra cash.

This last item might be held by the Officer in Charge against such an emergency. Do not pack or prepare for a weekend holiday but do not for lack of foresight be short of these minor comforts which will make your difficulties more bearable. The less you have to look for and ask for when you are in a blitzed area, the more you will help everyone.

The service reached its peak of development during the latter months of 1942 and the early months of 1943 when about a 100,000 full-time firemen were employed, 30,000 firewomen and over 200,000 part-time personnel.

When Britain and her Allies began planning for the eventual assault against occupied Europe, there was a gradual shift from passive defence to an offensive strategy, with budgets and manpower being diverted to meet this need. The Civil Defence Service was reduced in manpower, with eventual changes being made to the staffing and manpower levels of the NFS. Firefighting services were transferred to local authorities under the Fire Services Bill of 1947, which was enacted in 1948. The pre-war figure of over a thousand fire brigades was reduced, by the Bill, to 146 brigade authorities.

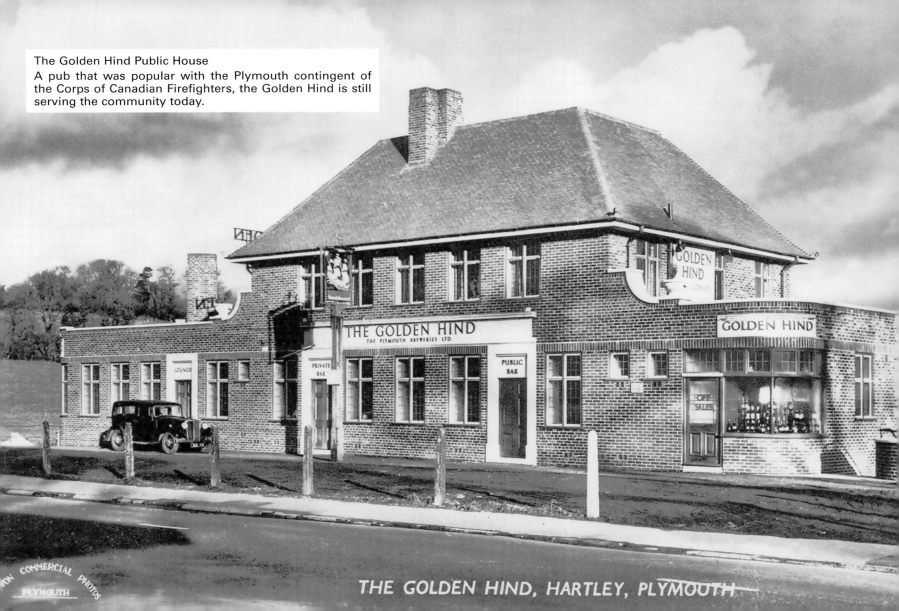

The Golden Hind Public House

A pub that was popular with the Plymouth contingent of the Corps of Canadian Firefighters, the Golden Hind is still serving the community today.

THE GOLDEN HIND, HARTLEY, PLYMOUTH

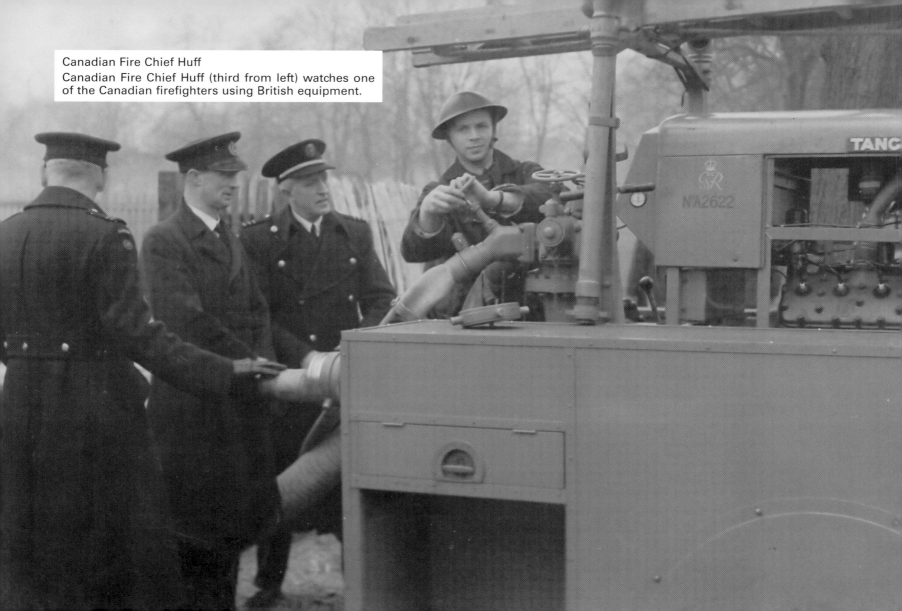

Canadian Fire Chief Huff
Canadian Fire Chief Huff (third from left) watches one of the Canadian firefighters using British equipment.

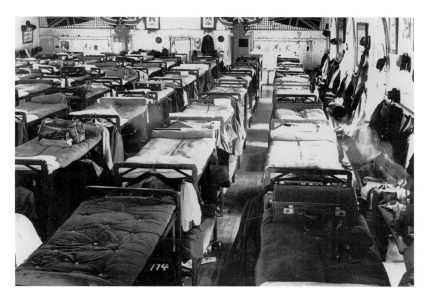

Firefighters' Messing Room
Above: One of the messing rooms for the firefighters, believed to be in Plymouth.

Training
Right: Ladder drill and firefighting training on a mocked-up building.

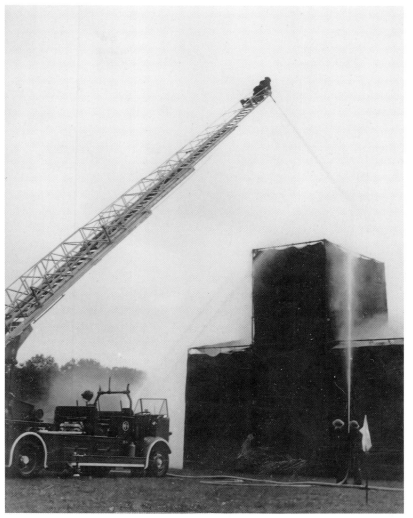

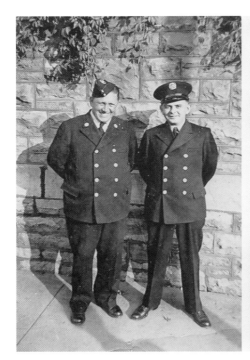
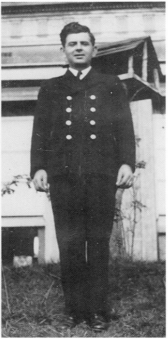

Personal Photos of Corps Members
Left: Officers who travelled to England. They have not yet been identified.

Horseplay
Right: This is some sort of firefighters' 'ritual': the original caption reads 'horseplay'!

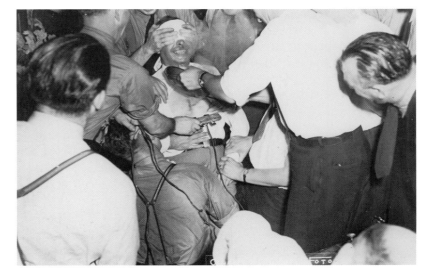

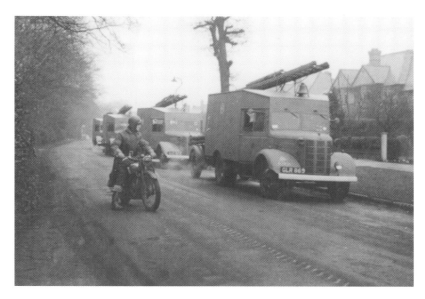

Leisure Time I
Left: Firefighters off duty in the messing hall.

Leisure Time II
Right: NFS convoy with which the Canadians would have become familiar.

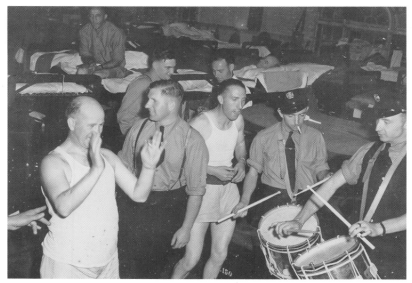

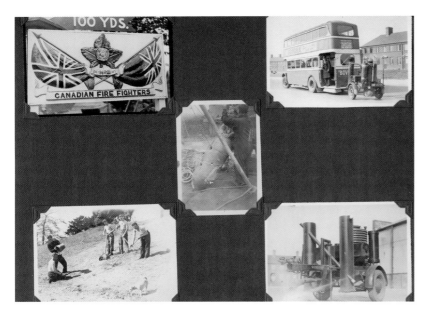

Plymouth I
Right: Plymouth after a raid, 1942.

Personal Snaps (Poly-Photos)
Left: Personal photographs, which were taken in England, showing an unexploded bomb, a bus with gas supply for fuel and firemen at play.

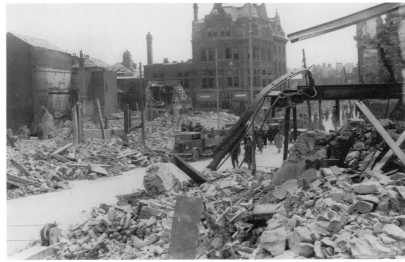

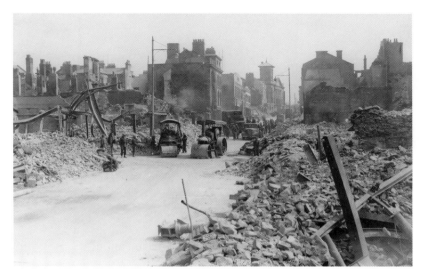

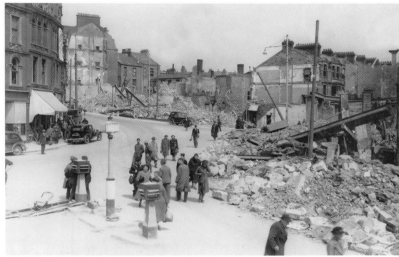

Above: Plymouth, Location Unknown I

Above right: Plymouth, Location Unknown II

New Turntable Ladder
Below right: Inspecting a new turntable ladder: this is a Merryweather.

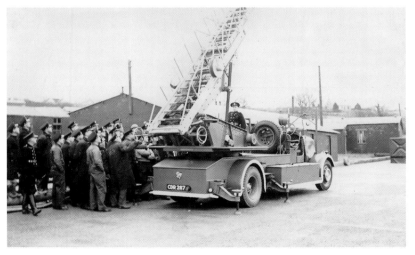

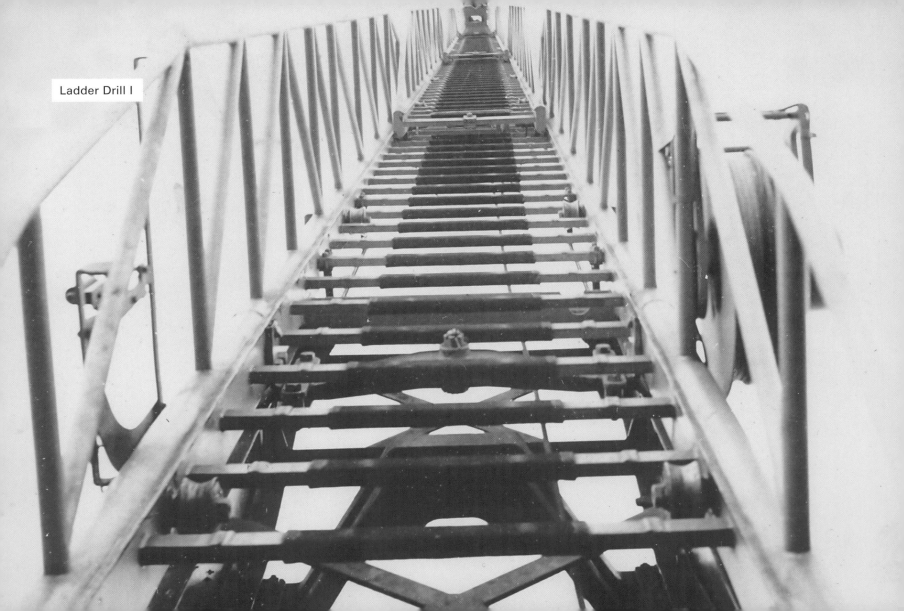

Ladder Drill I

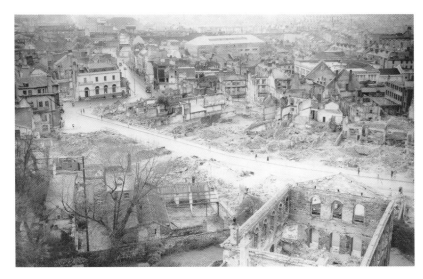

Plymouth

Right: This Plymouth scene, the exact location unknown, was used for training classes and for recording the activities of the Corps under fire.

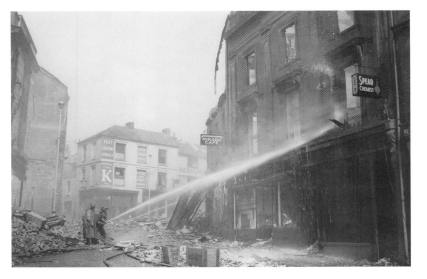

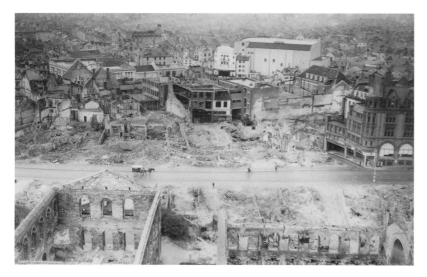

Plymouth Street Scene
Right: The aftermath of a raid with site clearance underway

Left: Another view of the city after enemy raids.

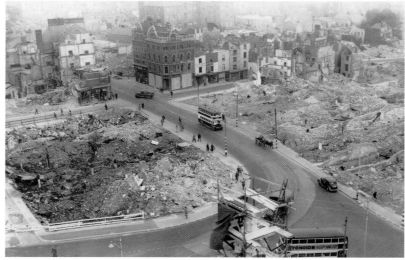

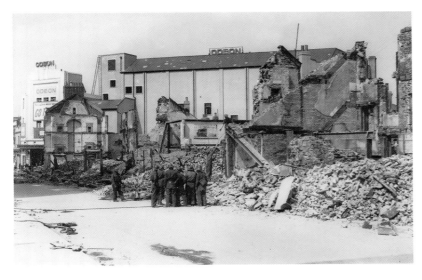

Above and right: Plymouth

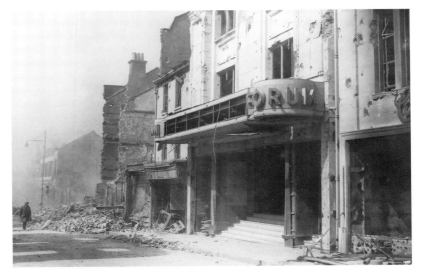

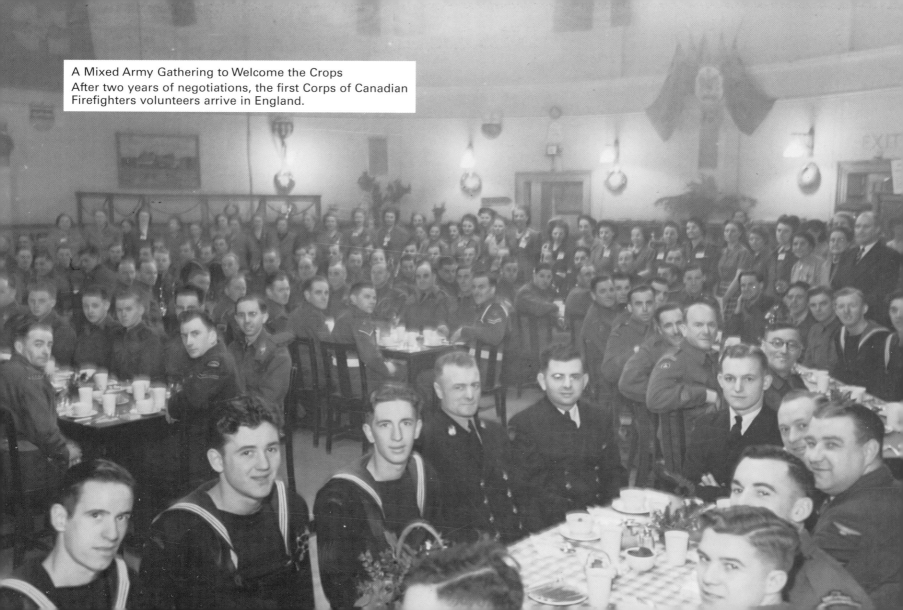

A Mixed Army Gathering to Welcome the Crops
After two years of negotiations, the first Corps of Canadian
Firefighters volunteers arrive in England.

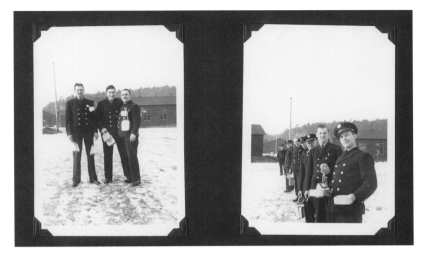

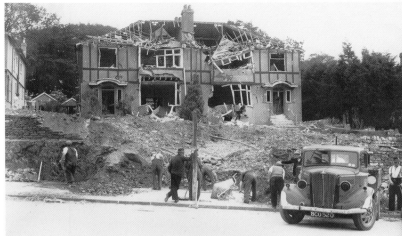

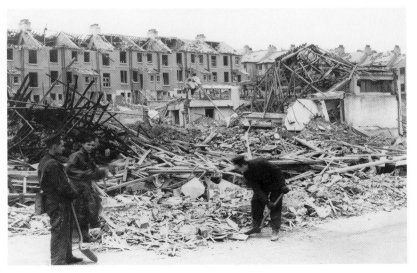

Personal Photos
Above: Winter time at Ivy bridge.

Plymouth Blitzed
Right: Two images taken following air raids on Plymouth. 'When we arrived we saw the people streaming up the hill to the caves outside the city.'

5

ALL FOR ONE AND ONE FOR ALL

Having given up their safe existence in Canada to travel through U-boat infested waters to an uncertain future helping to fight fires on British soil under the conditions of a country at war, these volunteers excelled in their duties and left a lasting impression on all those with whom they served and all those they met during their time in England.

Within just two years from its mobilisation in September 1939, the peacetime Fire Service had, despite many operational problems and other related difficulties, met the challenges thrust upon it by war.

The 1938 peacetime strength of some 50,000 personnel had expanded, in its new civil defence role, from 200,000 at the outbreak of war in 1939 to about 300,000 by the spring of 1941. The combined strength of the service comprised regular firemen, volunteers, part-timers and members of the AFS. In addition, there were civilian stirrup pump parties as well as various supplementary firefighting groups.

However, there was a need for more help. Bombing of English cities continued, and although there was a brief lull, in mid-1941 further significant attacks took place on London. The Fire Service had now been nationalised. A renewed call for assistance went out from the British government, and further consideration was given to the formation of a Canadian firefighting unit to serve in the United Kingdom.

Various meetings took place between and within the British and Canadian governments, where matters including pay, pension, benefits, transportation, recruitment, finance and equipment for and the actual status of the firefighters were discussed at length.

On 2 August 1941, the Canadian Secretary of the War Cabinet advised the Minister of National War Services that,

At a meeting of the Cabinet War Committee of 29 July, further consideration was given to the formation of a Canadian firefighting unit for service in the United Kingdom. In view of the recent reorganisation of the United Kingdom firefighting service and because of the purely civilian character of the force it was decided that the organisation of the proposed Canadian unit should be undertaken by the Department of National War Services rather than by the Department of National Defence as had first been contemplated.

In this connection it was agreed that an initial Canadian unit of from 400 to 500 men should be formed on the basis of the proposals which have been outlined in recent communications from the Canadian High Commissioner in London'.

From 24 June 1942 and for several months thereafter, a total of 406 volunteers in several contingents arrived in the United Kingdom and, after training and familiarisation, units were posted to major cities including, London, Bristol and Portsmouth. The Canadian volunteers served until the end of the war. They saw service during the continuation of the Blitz and were involved in various activities in support of the preparations for the D-Day landings.

From reports they had received about the bombing of British towns and cities, Canadian firefighters were in fact keen to support their English colleagues as early as 1940. A leading advocate for this was Lieutenant-Colonel Lister, who was then Chief of the Fire Service in British Columbia. Interestingly and independently, similar proposals had also been made by the fire services in Ontario and Manitoba. In London, severe enemy raids during the nights of 29 and 30 December 1940 indicated that there would be no let-up in the raids foreseeable into 1941. The British authorities were prompted to reconsider the support offered by the Canadians some time previously.

The Home Office drew up proposals for the recruitment, transportation and, accommodation of firefighters as well as training in the methods used by the NFS under wartime conditions. Included in the terms given for any assistance was that the Canadians were, for politically inspired reasons, to be regarded as civilians and as volunteers. It was determined by the British government that up to 1,000 trained firemen would be welcome. One of the unwritten agreements was that the Canadians would help to 'boost the morale' of both firefighters and the British population alike. They would be regarded as a valuable resource and as 'brothers in arms', standing shoulder to shoulder at a time of need.

Active recruiting did not begin until 11 March 1942, some two years after the offer of help was first proposed. It has been suggested that political wrangling, personality clashes between government officials and uncertainty as to how the Canadians could be deployed on the British mainland were contributory reasons for the delay. Following the selection and training of the firefighters in Canada, the volunteers embarked for England. The first contingent docked nine days later. It was June 1942, and on the 26th of that month a news despatch from London reported that twenty Canadian firemen had been taken on a tour of bomb-damaged sites in the city and in some of the outlying districts. Their guide was Sir Jocelyn Lucas, the welfare officer for Commonwealth troops in London. One fireman (later Leading Fireman) George Laskey (number T27), who hailed from Brantford, Ontario, commented to the media that 'We are all volunteers. A fire attracts a fireman like the sea attracts seamen so we are anxious to see the fire damage done in London.'

The official welcome ceremony for the advance contingents took place in Trafalgar Square, London, on 30 June, with Home

Secretary Herbert Morrison attending on behalf of the British government. In his welcome Morrison said,

> Now you come to add a new kind of contribution to the common effort. You come to play your part in our Blitzed cities, in the hazards and struggles in our fighting Home Front. When the day of trial comes again, as none of us forget that it may come with little warning, you will be here to meet and defeat its terrors.

A report in the *Brantford Expositer* newspaper of Canada in September (1942) stated that Commanding Officer G. E. Huff of the Corps of Canadian Fire Fighters and Fire Chief of the Brantford Fire Department had landed safely in England having travelled in a bomber of the RAF Ferry Command. (Huff was in fact 'on loan' from the Royal Canadian Air Force. He held the rank of Flight Lieutenant and was also the Fire Prevention Officer stationed with No. 2 RCAF Command at Winnipeg) On arrival he was met by officials of the NFS and by officers of the Corps who had preceded him to England. Huff's first duty was to inspect the five contingents of the Corps despatched overseas and their stations and billeting arrangements. It was expected that his tour would be brief and that upon his return to Canada, he would discuss with the Department of National War Services the set-up arrangements of the Canadian units.

During a banquet held in honour of Chief Officer Huff immediately prior to his visit to England, the Hon. J. T. Thorson, a Canadian government minister, said that 'Commander Huff will lead his men into a dangerous activity. They know it and know the job they will be called upon to do. In this I have every confidence that they will carry on in the best tradition of the Dominion (of Canada).' The Dominion Fire Chief Commissioner, W. L. Clairmont, added: 'We in Canada should be proud to have a Corps connected to the National Fire Service of Great Britain.'

The newspaper editorial concluded with a statement from Huff in which he said that 'Canada's new unit of overseas firemen who will battle incendiary blazes started by the Luftwaffe may soon be armed against low level machine gun attacks by Nazi fliers'. History tells us that this fortunately never happened.

The *Manchester Evening News*, one of the many regional papers that took up the story of the arrival and dispersal of the Canadians, wrote on 15 May 1943 that the Canadians were as 'A blood transfusion for a sorely wounded warrior'.

Cyril Kendall, an officer in the NFS, said, 'The Canadians donated thousands of feet of rubber hose which became known, not surprisingly as Canadian Hose. That was one of the best things that ever happened, getting all that hose which fitted and with the addition of our connectors could be used anywhere.'

The groups were dispersed according to perceived need as soon as training was complete. Corps Headquarters was situated in Inner Park Road, Wimbledon, London, close to Wimbledon Common. It comprised the administrative offices for the Corps in England, with stores as well as accommodation for officers and other ranks on a site that also had a number of connecting huts. The principal officers of the Corps were supported here by staff including clerks, cooks and drivers. Joyce Lewis was an NFS driver from 1941: 'The Canadians, yes I remember them well. They fought with us in London and they had a station at Wimbledon later on. Nice lads they were and they went through the thick of it.'

Detachment 1 was sent to Southampton and arrived there in August 1942, with the men being divided between the stations in Hulse Road and Marsh Lane, commanded by Chief Officer Thornton and Chief Officer Scott respectively. In this city the Canadians helped with the provision of static water tanks, but crucially assisted the NFS during the trials of the PLUTO pipeline which ran off Lepe Beach just a short distance from the mouth of Southampton Water. Lepe is now a country park managed by Hampshire County Council.

Tom Porter, who was serving as a member of the NFS, recalls,

I first met the Canadians when our unit was moved to Testwood. We had always drawn most of our fuel from Testwood before we were transferred there although we also had access to a pump on a local garage forecourt and when the Canadians arrived we went with them to draw fuel from the garage.

May Belbin, an NFS firewomen, remembers,

The Canadians came to Southampton, I don't know how many, but there were quite a few. They used to tell us about their families because I suppose they were homesick which is quite understandable, but also it helped us to get to know them better and they became part of our big family.

Detachment 2 served Plymouth, with the first group of men arriving there in September 1942 after a period of training at Lee Mill, Ivybridge, Devon. A second group of Canadians arrived in January 1943, and this brought the total contingent strength there to seventy-four men.

Tom Adams recalls,

I remember the firefighters well because being a young apprentice in heating and hot water work, I was involved on building work in Tor Lane, Hartley in Plymouth. This building was for the Canadians when they came over here to help the National Fire Service.

There was a crest of the door of the station with a motto which read 'All For One and One For All'. I was about fourteen at that time and it was part of life in the war. Seeing new people, and the Canadians, well they were a nice crowd of chaps and very friendly to everyone.

Phyllis Wilshaw (née Dilling) from Plymouth remembers,

I was sent to the Fire Service in 1943, and was based with the Canadians at Hartley in Plymouth. My duty meant that I did one night a week with this great group of chaps. There was always plenty of food available and it wasn't rationed like it was for civilians. Until about 1944, I courted one of the men, he was Section Leader Frank Dymond, but I was then called up to serve with the ATS.

The Canadians were well known and very popular in the area and when they had dances every so often, everyone turned up.

Fire stations in Greenbank Road and Victoria Road were the initial bases for the men, although just six months later, in March 1943, a new austerity-built ten-bay station was opened at The Drive in Hartley close to Tor House, the accommodation centre for the Plymouth detachment. The Canadians had by then experienced enemy air raids on the city, the first being in January of 1943 when high explosives were dropped on the outskirts. Another heavy attack was experienced over a one-and-a-half hour period on 13 February, when both high explosives and incendiaries were dropped on the city.

Bristol was the location of Detachment 3, with some eighty personnel being accommodated at Stoke House in the grounds of Clifton Theological College on the north-west outskirts of the city.

Dennis Perrett of Bristol remembers,

I was aged ten when the Canadians came and we used to scrounge chocolate from them. Their station was on Stoke Hill in an old building known as the Theological Hall, near Durham Downs.

After the war I visited the Hall when I was then in the building trade. The firemen had carved their names in the lead which was covering the three 'domes' of the building.

Reg Weekes recalled,

I was a Section Leader in the National Fire Service stationed on the old premises of the Bristol Motor Company in Victoria Street. It was from there that we were sent on a refresher course to a camp near Ivybridge in Devon where me and the others first met and became friendly with several Canadians who came with their different uniforms and accents to be with us during those difficult times. I seem to recall being with them again during the Second Front when we were then stationed in Southampton. Although there were by now more of these fun-loving men and then suddenly they were gone and out of our lives and we all wondered 'Where are they now?'

One of the major incidents attended by the Canadians was a ship fire in Avonmouth Docks when there was an explosion aboard the SS Massachusetts. This ship was carrying oil and ammunition, and the resulting fire also involved a hundred NFS personnel and two fireboats.

Ruth Davies was doing compulsory duty at the same station as the Canadians: 'There were about a hundred Canadian firemen stationed here and their chief was called Lambert. At Athenaeum Street we used to gather at a club for coffee and a chat. No alcohol of course. After the war five local girls married five of the Canadian chaps.'

In early 1944, the Germans dropped high explosives, incendiaries and phosphorous bombs over a wide area of Somerset to the south of Bristol and the entire Corps contingent was instrumental in saving a large part of the stores at the Royal Army Ordnance Corps depot at Weave in Somerset. In the same county, near Taunton, the United States had its Southern Command depot, which was used for the supply of general stores, clothing and food to the US forces stationed across the south-west of England. As the build up to D-Day intensified, the resident US Army firefighting section was withdrawn from the depot and was prepared for going into Europe. So it came about that sixteen firemen, a section leader and three leading firemen with a company officer from the Corps of Canadian Firefighters were assigned to duty at the depot.

In November 1942, Detachment 4 of the Corps arrived in the south coast city of Portsmouth, where they were greeted and inspected by the Lord Mayor before taking up their duties at stations in Craneswater Avenue and Auckland Road East.

Accommodation was provided nearby at the Clarence Hotel and at Craneswater Park.

Jennifer Turner remembers:

Mother was a widow when I was young so it was not improper that she took up the offer of going to local dances with one of the Canadians. I am sorry but I do not know his name. All the men I met were good to me as a child and gave me small gifts usually consisting of some of their rations which included sweets. My mother said that they used to talk a lot about their families and that they always acted like real gentlemen. I believe some of the men used to get invited to people's homes for meals but I can't be sure. I know that one of the firemen was killed in the city, but I only found that out after the war when the story was told to me by an aunt.

The heavy enemy raid on Portsmouth on 15 and 16 August 1943 resulted in the Canadians dealing with many of the seventy or so fires started by the bombing, and when the enemy carried out further scattered raids on the city in early 1944, the Corps was on continuous duty over several nights.

Off duty, the Canadians excelled at team competitions. Jack Coulter recalls,

We had a tow vehicle and trailer pump and we would have to drive forward to a tank. The idea was to disconnect the pump from the truck then get the suction in the water of the tank, lay the hose out and knock down a target with the jet of water. This was a fairly standard type of competition. We Canadians probably being a little younger and a little more active than the

British were able to compete well and we became the winners of the competition. As a result we were presented with a trophy. All this was filmed by a crew from Canada working for the National Film Board.

May Belbin recalls: 'We used to have field [sports] days and for that I used to wear my best uniform. We went and served teas from the mobile kitchen that had been donated by the Canadian Red Cross.'

Tom Porter also remembers field days attended by the Canadians,

The thing that struck me was the strength of these men. They were very strong and could pick up a light pump off its trailer and carry it without any trouble. There were handles on the end for the British firemen to lift the pump. Also another thing that struck me was the way they handled fire gear. When they ran out a hose they never carried the branch (hose) under their arm like we did. They just threw it from one man to the next a bit like throwing a baseball.

Although by this time, air attacks on Britain had begun to diminish, the Canadians saw service during calls to both major incidents and lull period incidents. Subsequent to the Normandy Campaign and following an agreement between the Canadian and British governments, demobilisation began in late 1944 when the National War Services Department announced plans for the first group to leave. Remaining groups would leave as stations were closed. The official announcement stated that conditions no longer made it necessary to maintain the Corps as protection against enemy attacks, and while some Corps members had volunteered to serve on the continent there was insufficient grounds for them to do so. About two-thirds of the Corps were firefighters in civilian life, and it was expected their experiences would prove beneficial when they returned to their own communities. The British authorities had arranged a number of farewell ceremonies to express appreciation of the contribution made by the Corps.

Colonel J. W. Dear, who hailed from Ottawa, was to stay behind with a small staff to clear up all the administrative tasks as the Corps members departed. It was he who organised the gift of CAD $38,000-worth of the Corps clothing and equipment to the National Fire Service 'in appreciation of the training and assistance received by the Corps in Britain'.

The British government later announced that members of the Corps who had served in Britain for a year or more would be entitled to wear the Defence of Britain Medal. On behalf of the Canadian government, War Services Minister Dr McCann responded by saying that the medal ribbon would be made available immediately to all eligible former Corps members

Davina Stevens (née Simpson) from Brantford, Ontario, says: 'When I was at the Brantford Collegiate College in the early 1950s, our chemistry teacher Mr Brown used to regale us with stories of his time in London during the war when he used to stand on the roofs of buildings waiting to put out incendiary fires.'

During their service on Britain's Home Front, the Canadians suffered five casualties and three deaths. Fireman J. S. Coull, No. T112 of Winnipeg, died in July 1944, a casualty of a flying bomb attack. He is laid to rest in Scotland and at his burial he was given full military honours. Section Leader Lawrence 'Curly' Woodhead, No. T305, was from Saskatoon: he died in June 1944 when he fell from a speeding fire engine during a training exercise in Southampton. May Belbin again: 'They used to go out on manoeuvres and sometimes the fire engines were overloaded with men. One of the firemen fell off the lorry and was killed. They put his coffin in the hall and it was draped with the Canadian flag. We all went down to pay our respects.' Section Leader Alfred LaPierre, No. T212 of Montreal, died in Bristol in April 1943, and with Mr Woodhead was laid to rest in the grounds of the Canadian section of Brookwood Cemetery, Woking. Small flags of Canada are placed at the headstones and are renewed when weather-worn.

The ship that transported many of the Corps of Canadian Fire Fighters to Liverpool was no ordinary vessel, and as such it is worthy of a mention. Among seafaring folk there is a belief that some ships are jinxed and others are lucky. The Dominion Monarch fell into the latter category … but there is an ironic twist to the tale.

Constructed in 1938 at the Swan Hunter shipyard on Tyneside, in the north of England, the motor ship (or MV as it was designated) had a displacement of just over 27,000 tons and a speed of 21½ knots. She became the flagship of the Shaw Savill Line and was one of the sleekest and most admired vessels of her type. The Shaw Savill Line was a firmly established shipping company, having been founded in the nineteenth century. Upon launch, the Dominion Monarch was the largest ship sailing to Australia and New Zealand. She was almost at the end of her initial outward bound journey when war was declared, and hurried plans were made to arm her upon arrival at her port of destination. Unfortunately there were very few guns available in Australia, but great ingenuity was shown in strengthening the isolation hospital and other areas of the ship in preparation for guns and mountings to be installed.

The homeward bound journey was uneventful until the ship reached the River Thames. Her arrival coincided with the discovery of the first magnetic mines laid by the Germans at the mouth of the river, yet the Dominion Monarch managed to avoid these and arrived safely at the King George V Dock in the Port of London. Fred Cook was born in the East End of London and remembers: 'Her arrival would be announced by an ear-splitting roar of her siren. Being a motor vessel, the siren used compressed air which resounded far and wide.'

On her return from that voyage, she was surveyed for possible service as a transport ship, but in 1939 the authorities had not envisaged the large-scale conversions needed, which were later to become the standard. It was on the grounds that her luxurious passenger accommodation would prevent her carrying more than a comparatively small number of troops that she was rejected at that time. She had an uneventful second wartime voyage running with few passengers and much empty cargo space, but on her return journey she was used for the stowage of foodstuffs which did not require refrigeration. At Cape Town she filled her fuel tanks to capacity, and this provided an excess of 600 tons, which she landed in London to assist in meeting the nation's demand for oil.

In 1940, the need for ships of all types for war service was becoming a priority, and the Dominion Monarch was finally requisitioned by the government in August of that year. She became the first ship to be converted into a troopship, and this was completed in Liverpool. The areas that previously accommodated five hundred passengers were, after conversion, able to accommodate 142 officers and 1,300 other ranks, although there was still far more space available in this large vessel.

During her post-conversion trip to Australia via Port Said, where the full complement of troops was disembarked, the Dominion Monarch went into dry dock at Cockatoo Island so that work to strengthen her anti-aircraft defences could be completed before the homeward voyage. It was becoming apparent that the sea lanes were becoming more dangerous by the day and more vulnerable to enemy attack. Upon her return to Liverpool, the ship was surprisingly transferred back to the Liner Requisition Scheme, but almost immediately this was overruled and she remained a Transport under what was known as the T97A Agreement.

On a later voyage, the ship took reinforcements out to Singapore; they were landed at the time that the Japanese Army was advancing ever closer to the island. The situation in the region was becoming more critical by the hour. Despite this, and rather curiously, the ship was ordered to dry dock to have her engines overhauled. As she lay in the dock, partially dismantled, air attacks by the Japanese became more intense, and most of the labour force in the dockyard had already fled. However, undaunted, the chief engineer and crew were able to get the engines into working order, and they steered the ship away from the port just before the Japanese finally overran the island. Dominion Monarch made a run for New Zealand, where she arrived safely before a voyage home via the Panama Canal. That alone more than endorsed her reputation as a lucky ship.

Again back at her home port, the ship was subject to modifications that provided extra capacity for troops, and the numbers she could accommodate crept up from around the original 1,500 to well in excess of four thousand by the end of her war service. For a large and conspicuous ship, the Dominion Monarch was indeed lucky to avoid the wolf packs of German submarines as well as attack by sea and air. During the 350,000 miles she travelled, the ship carried nearly 90,000 people. Some of these were German prisoners of war being transported to America, but for the most part the ship carried Armed Services personnel of the Commonwealth. The commander, chief steward and chief engineer were all awarded honours by His Majesty King George VI.

In the late 1940s and early 1950s, the ship was one of several vessels which participated in the £10 assisted passage scheme that allowed British emigrants to travel to Australia and New Zealand. The Dominion Monarch was used as a floating hotel at the legendary 1962 World's Fair in Seattle, made famous by the film *It Happened* at the World's Fair starring Elvis Presley. Ironically, after escaping the enemy invasion of Singapore, the ship ended her life in Japanese ownership as the Dominion Monarch Maru, and she was unceremoniously scrapped later in 1962.

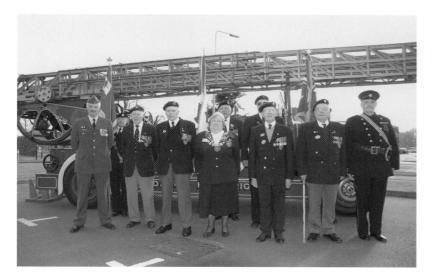

Above: Canadian representatives and veterans at the dedication ceremony.

Right: Possibly en route to the Testwood Training Centre, a member of the Crops adopts a Winston Churchill 'victory sign'.

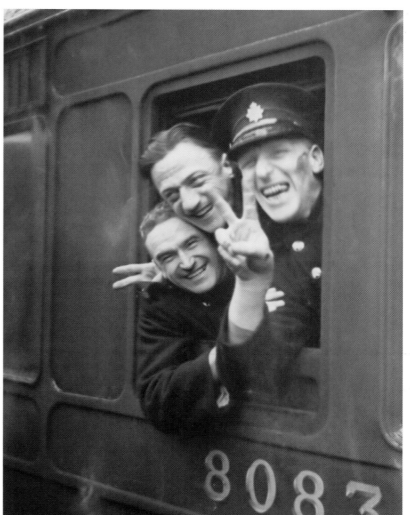

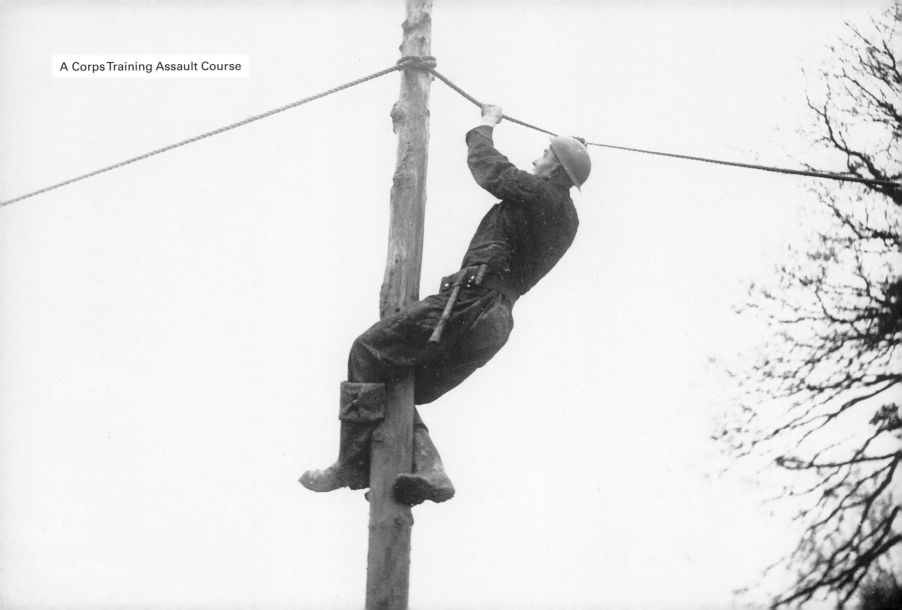

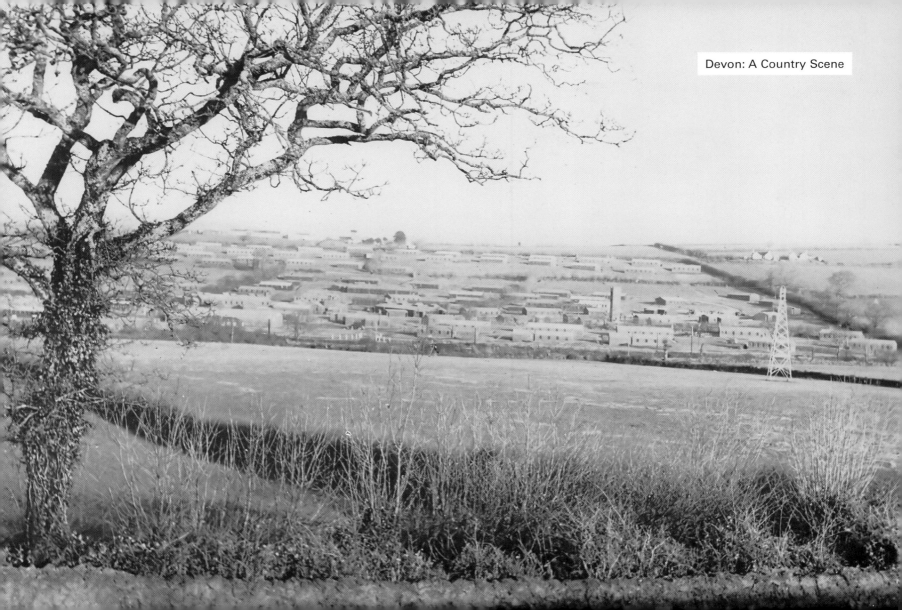

Devon: A Country Scene

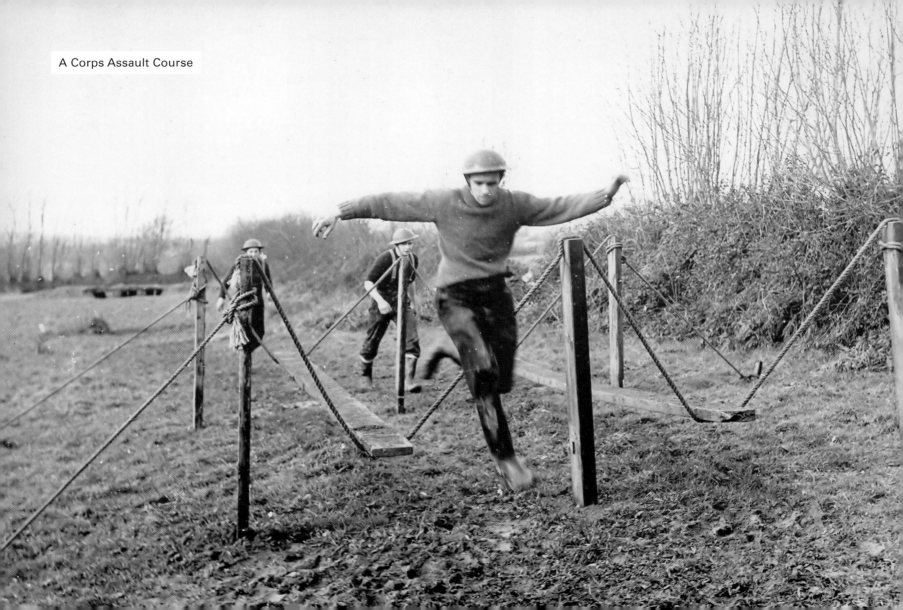

A Corps Assault Course

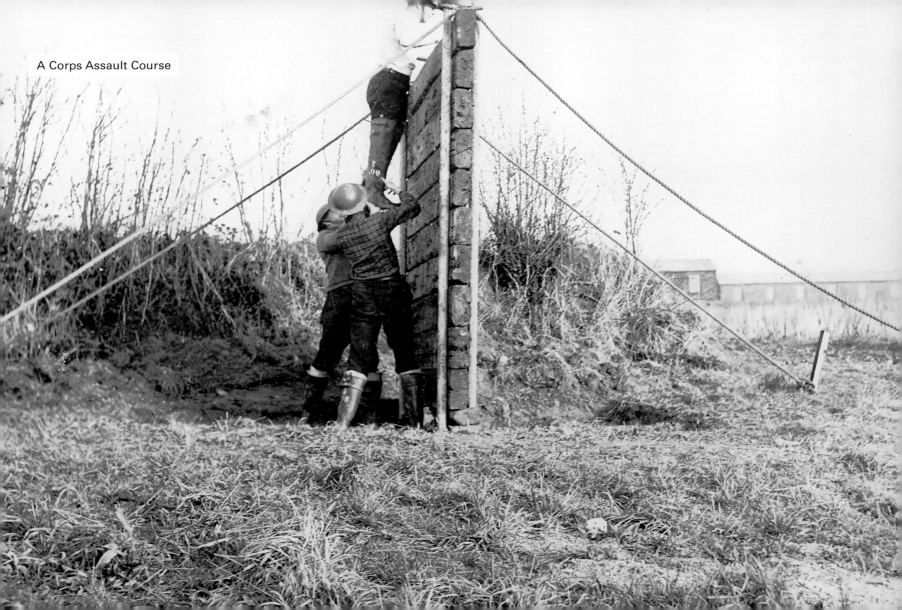

A Corps Assault Course

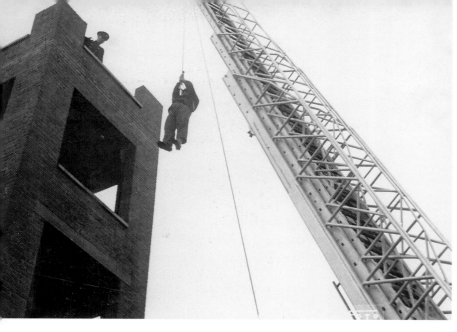

Right: Hose-laying Drill

Left: Ladder Drill I

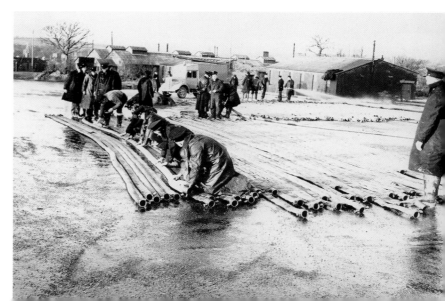

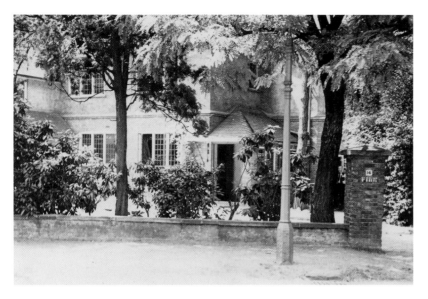

Right: Tor House

Left: Two views of Tor House at Hartley which was requisitioned for use by the Plymouth Contingent.

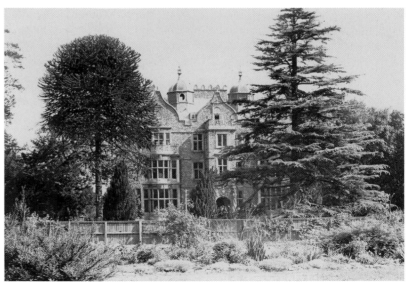

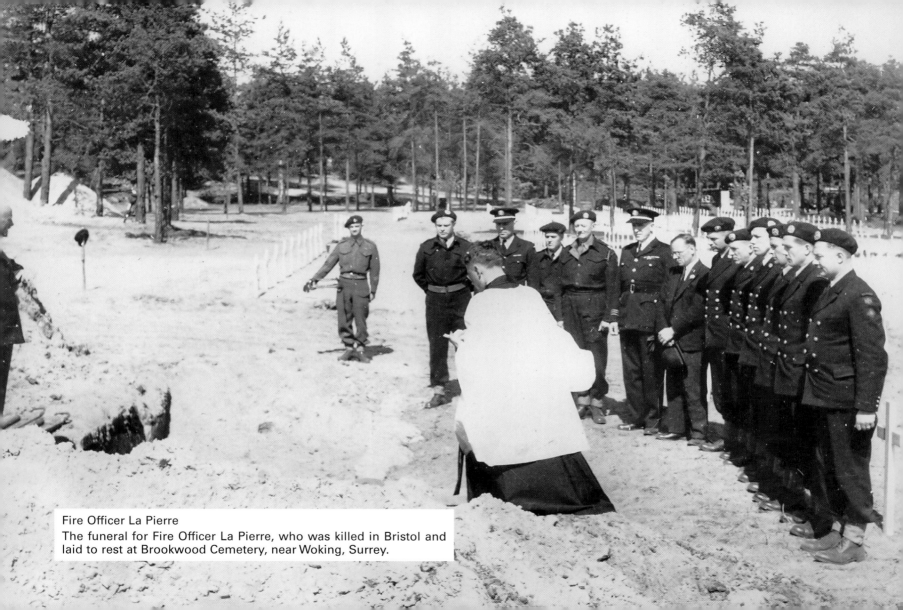

Fire Officer La Pierre
The funeral for Fire Officer La Pierre, who was killed in Bristol and laid to rest at Brookwood Cemetery, near Woking, Surrey.

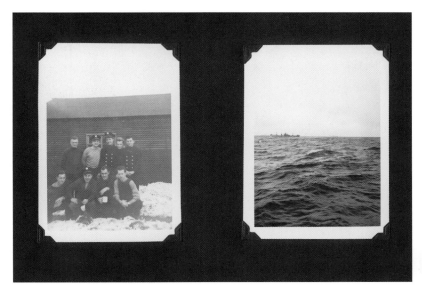

Personal Photos
Right: A selection of personal keepsake photographs of Corps members.

Personal Photos
Left: A selection of personal keepsake photographs of Corps members.

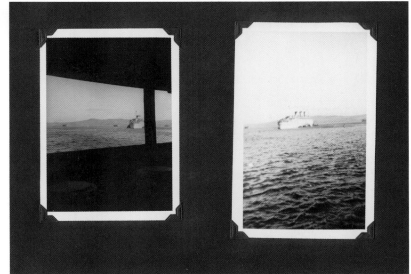

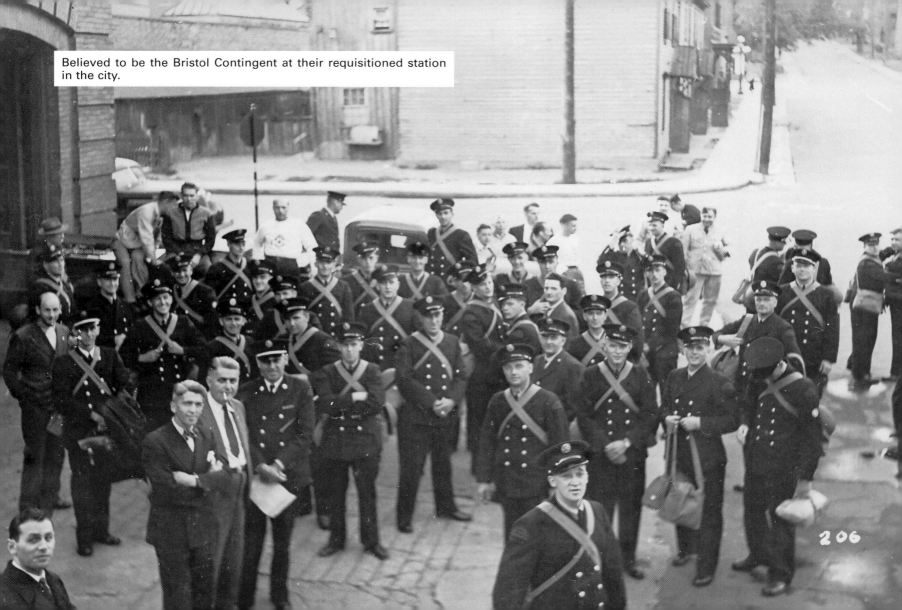

Believed to be the Bristol Contingent at their requisitioned station in the city.

206

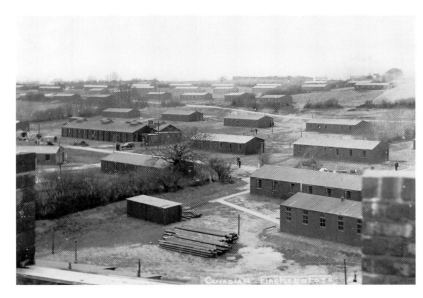

Fire Service Camp

Right: A depot/training area somewhere in the south of England; the exact location is unknown.

Left: Personal Photos

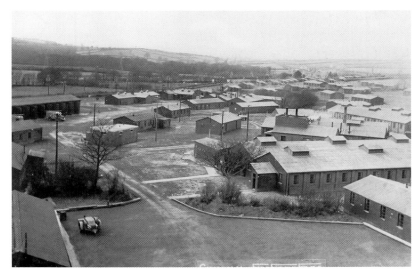

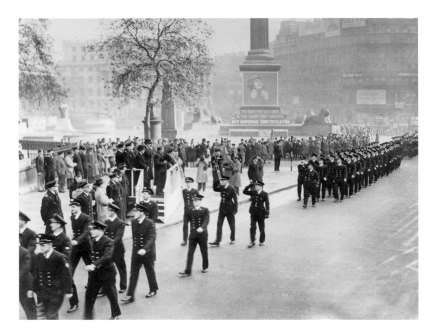

The Corps of Canadian Firefighters Arrive

Right and above: After two years of negotiations, the first Corps of Canadian Firefighters volunteers arrive in England.

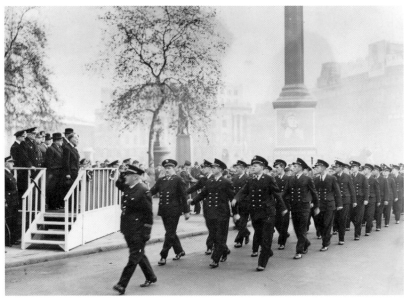

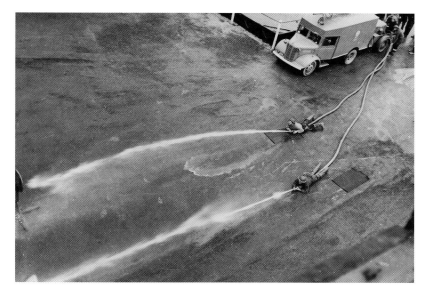

Fire Appliance
Above: Training with hoses, despite their full workload the men were learning new techniques all the time.

New Appliances
Right: New appliances issued to the Plymouth contingent.

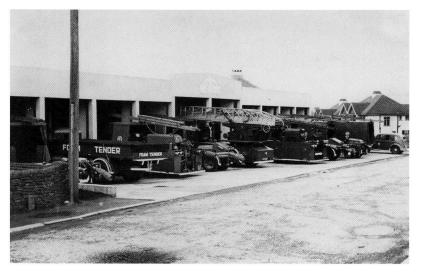

BROTHERS IN ARMS

Canada's Prime Minister Mackenzie King embarked on a special mission to Great Britain in 1941 at the request of the British government. Subsequent to that meeting it was agreed that Canada would form an organisation called the Corps of Canadian Firefighters which would be sent overseas for service alongside the NFS in England. The organisation would be under the direction of the Minister of National War Service.

Fire Chief D. A. Boulden of Winnipeg was selected to lead the Corps, and later in 1941 he moved to Ottawa for the purpose of planning and setting up the unit. However, for reasons that remain unclear to this day, he left Ottawa in January 1942 and Fire Chief G. E. Huff of the city of Brantford in south-western Ontario took over as commanding officer. It was two months later in March 1942 that recruitment began.

Jack Coulter was typical of the men who trained for firefighting duties in England. When an appeal went out to the Army Fire Service personnel in Canada for volunteers for overseas service with the newly formed Corps of Canadian Firefighters, Coulter was among the first to offer his support for his comrades in England. He became a Leading Fireman No. T74, and his story is told through personal interviews and transcriptions of his own personal diary notes as well as archive research.

Jack began by saying,

I was one of sixteen volunteers from the Winnipeg Fire Department reacting in response to the call to serve in Britain. At the time of enlistment I was stationed at No. 3 Station on a temporary basis, but I had been talking to colleagues Bill Carr, Alex Smith and Bill Neill over at No. 1 Station for some time about the opportunity of going overseas and in fact we sent our applications into Ottawa at the same time. We had to resign from the Fire Service at home and my letter, a copy of which I kept for my family, is dated May 6th 1942. Alex Smith and I took the week's leave we were permitted before embarkation and as Alex had just married Jean McDonald, daughter of a fire captain, this week was a sort of honeymoon as well.

When we arrived in Ottawa, the first contingent of about fifty officers and men were already partly through their identification, uniform and kit processing. I was part of a second contingent of fifty men and officers so by the time we got to our temporary accommodation on the third floor of an old fire hall [station] in Lower Town it was rather cramped. So we slept in three-tier bunks and had very small washroom facilities, just the basics.

We were in Ottawa for about three weeks doing not much more than marching around the area near the fire hall during the day which I supposed kept us fit. We had the film people down from Canadian National Film [National Film Board of Canada] and they had the cameras rolling as we went through various marching and exercises. Later they came over to England to complete the film which was released to cinema audiences in Canada after the war.

At night Jack and his fellow firefighters found cheap places to eat and they visited numerous bars, including the Standish Hall Hotel. Jack remembers this had the longest bar he had ever seen. Owned by J. P. Maloney, the venue had been converted into a nightclub, but was, as fate would have it, destroyed by fire in 1951.

Jack continued,

When we had been kitted out we were given one week's embarkation leave as I mentioned before, with a return train ticket home. At home we had our pictures in the local newspapers and we were given a great send off by the community when we left. We arrived back in Ottawa and it wasn't long before we boarded a train for Halifax, Nova Scotia. Our ship, the Motor Vessel Dominion Monarch was already loaded with several thousand servicemen before we embarked. This was quite a fast ship because it was new, having been built in 1938 by Swan Hunter for the Shaw Savill Line. I believe it was requisitioned as a troopship in about 1940 so the crew, by the time we boarded, were well used to the needs of the military in wartime.

During the crossing of the Atlantic enemy submarines were spotted and we would then manoeuvre at speed on a changed course so that the escort destroyers could clear the area with depth charges. I was told that the speed of our ship was in excess of 20 knots which was enough to outrun German U-boats at that time, thank goodness. The *Dominion Monarch* was a refrigerator ship in part with the rest of the areas left for conversion to a troop carrier. She was on a return trip to England from Australia so had crossed many dangerous waters already before we embarked. I understand she had almost been captured by the Japanese during the fall of Singapore in February 1942.

Quarters for us were below deck at the bow end and they were accessed by a very steep ladder. We were offered mutton to eat, but I couldn't stand it so opted for just plain bread and cheese with occasional jam for my meals throughout the entire nine-day journey. I was missing my mother's home cooking as I am sure most lads were who were taking this adventure overseas.

The British government had asked for up to a thousand volunteers, but the total strength was 422 men – some of whom were based at headquarters in Canada. They were recruited from all provinces of the Dominion of Canada. From completion of training and preparation through to December 1942, when the last Canadian contingent arrived in England, these men were left in no doubt as to what lay ahead of them.

We arrived in Liverpool [Jack continues], and then we were taken by train to the Testwood area of Totton just outside the city of

Southampton on the south coast. What I saw of the English countryside during that journey over many hours made me quite fall in love with the place. At Testwood, which was a converted school run by the National Fire Service, we were given a four-week course on firefighting under wartime conditions and rescue work, and we also did a lot of drill.

We were instructed on the trailer pumps, they were either Coventry Climax or Dennis pumps I remember, and we laid out the hose one length at a time instead of laying the hose out from the back of a hose wagon as we had been used to back home.

The pumps we mostly used had a 500 gallon capacity and we had to start the four-cylinder petrol engine with a crank handle. I guess the whole unit was about 12 feet long and on the side was space for four lengths of rolled-up hose. Our towing vehicles for the pumps were Morrises and Austins, and the body was open to the rear with seating for up to six crew members and the vehicles were also equipped with lengths of 2½ inch rubber-lined hose with quick couplers for easy connection.

Practice with the equipment on the huge field at Testwood included trying to knock down targets at distance after having laid out the hose one length at a time, then attaching the nozzle. To be honest, so much time was spent in laying hose before any practice firefighting could begin.

After familiarisation training, the Corps was split up and sent for service in Portsmouth, Plymouth, Bristol and Southampton. Our headquarters unit was based in Wimbledon, London.

The second contingent of which I was a member was transferred into Southampton city and we were billeted in the Alliance Hotel [this was home to the Canadians for three years] just one block away from the entrance to the docks on the corner of Oxford Street and Latimer Street. The building still stands to this day. This hotel seemed a small place to us with three storeys and rooms facing front, to one side and to the rear. Living quarters were very sparse really, with a wood-frame bed and thin cotton-filled mattresses, a wooden locker and chair for each crew member, and we had one chest of drawers to share in each four-man room. In our room was Alex Smith, Stewart McMullen from Ottawa who lost a leg in a train accident when he returned to Canada, Joe Tennant who was from Kirkland Lake and me, Jack Coulter. Anyway, one good thing, the food was good in the wartime circumstances. Tom Kendall was a Canadian and in charge of the English cooks. Tom always got his supplies from a Canadian Forces supply base so we did all right.

There was a large dining room, like a large mess, and we all sat down together to eat. We also had a lounge and a piano, and quite by luck there were two great pianists among our team so sing-songs were very popular especially at Christmas time.

Our equipment was garaged in an old showroom of a nearby Daimler garage which our crew shared with the National Fire Service guys. There was space here enough for twenty vehicles with trailer pumps, and these were backed up against the perimeter walls. In the centre were specialised vehicles like the hose layers and salvage trucks and the larger pumps which the NFS men crewed.

When we walked to and from the garage, we had to pass four pubs: The Grapes in Oxford Street [still standing], The Bristol, The Castle, Trent Road [now a supermarket] and The Fox and Hounds, and it was interesting how each place had its own types of customer and its own unique atmosphere. Needless to say that we all became very good friends with the publicans!

The city of Southampton had the best docks we had seen and certainly the best in the south of England. It was said that the Germans wanted to use these facilities in the event they invaded. Most of the bomb damage had occurred before we arrived and we saw great damage in the downtown area, but I think the railway station and the city offices were hardly damaged.

One operational date that stuck in our minds was 19 August 1942 when we were sent over to Portsmouth, because this was after the Dieppe fiasco when the Germans repelled attacks by many Canadian servicemen and the wounded were being brought up from the docks in Portsmouth for transit to a relief camp. We firefighters felt pretty insignificant when we saw the wounded and bloodied soldiers. There had been much loss of Canadian life at Dieppe and many of our guys were taken prisoner.

On a much lighter note, sport was one of the most enjoyable and popular activities among Jack and his colleagues, and they played soccer with and against whomever they could find as opponents. Two of the Southampton contingent, friends Reg and Bill, were manager and coach, and as Jack says, they always managed to field a pretty good team,

A few of us were able to practise with the Southampton professional team and I used to hang out with the baseball team and was able to get many trips to other areas when we played both Canadian and American services teams. I really enjoyed that leisure-time activity. We also used to be good when competing in competitions with the National Fire Service and we won a special trophy. That occasion was captured on film and the trophy itself is still held in high esteem today here in Canada by our modern firemen and women. I know that particular day at Testwood, the mobile canteen was very well supported. One of the best visits away I remember was when we went over to Bournemouth. What a nice place and very cosmopolitan at the time with service personnel from all parts of the world. Fortunately this town did not suffer too much damage so a great relief for all the folk who lived there.

We had periods of leave, and we usually went up to Scotland because our friend Alex had relatives in Edinburgh and Aberdeen. The usual practice was to call in on a local fire station and stay there while we were away from the home base. I also remember we went to visit an aunt of Alex in Windsor, Berkshire, and we always tried to take some supplies from our base kitchen so we didn't have to impose on her meagre rations. When we were in London, we usually slept in a fire station just off the Strand.

Later in the war, the summer of 1944, when things were turning in favour of the Allies, we in Southampton were volunteering as life guards for the local swimming pool. Without us providing the staff, the kids in the neighbourhood lost out because the pool could not open.

For us it was difficult just to wait for the outcome of what was happening on the continent so we volunteered to serve with the British Army firefighters. It soon became clear we were not required for duty, and by now we had been told that we would be going home in December.

In fact, it was just after New Year 1945 dawned that we were embarking on the Mauritania at the port of Liverpool having been shipped up from the south coast. The voyage to Halifax,

Nova Scotia, was much better than the trip over and we were only five days getting back to Canada. On arrival we were whisked off the ship and onto a train for Ottawa where, believe it or not we ended up at the same fire hall. Following medical examinations and demobilisation we returned to Winnipeg where we were met by our families.

It was a marvellous feeling to be back home, it was almost like a dream.

Jack later wrote: 'We returned home just after Christmas 1944. The food was much better and there was no threat of U-boats.'

Jack and his colleagues appeared in a film shot by one of the Corps members with equipment loaned by the National Film Board of Canada. *Firemen Go To War* was released in 1946 as a joint National Film Board of Canada and Department of National War Services production. During its brief seventeen-minute running time, the film portrayed to the government and people of that country not only the severity of the impact of war on Britain, but also the part played by the gallant 406 Canadian firemen who served overseas between 1942 and 1945.

Produced by W. A. Macdonald and narrated by Don Pringle, the film was shot on 16 mm Kodachrome colour film at a number of locations throughout England by Section Leader Young, the Corps photographer. Today it stands as a remarkable and fascinating example of a wartime documentary, primarily because of its matter-of-fact and dispassionate approach to the subject.

Especially poignant are the scenes filmed in Plymouth and the Devonport area after one of the most devastating raids on the city. They epitomise the devastation inflicted upon many towns and cities, and the assistance provided to the often overstretched NFS by the units from Canada.

The narrative for the film was recorded on 22 March 1946, and it is obvious the studio team did the best they could to work it in with the footage at their disposal. Rather repetitively, and somewhat laboriously, it tells the story of the Corps and how its members acclimatised themselves to service in wartime England.

Don Pringle narrates with a suitably paced but somewhat over-dramatic tone,

England under fire! The battle of the Blitz! A story of high explosive bombs that smashed whole blocks, of fire bombs that showered down by the thousands. To the men and women of Britain, war came as a red rain from the skies. Ruin, destruction and lurking danger became part of everyday life.

Here was a war in which the civilian stood in the front line. Among those who bore the heaviest brunt of the Blitz were the men of the NFS, Britain's wartime organisation of firefighters. Their casualties were heavy. They needed reinforcements – trained reinforcements – and the need was desperate.

The British government turned to Canada. Could the Dominion raise a Corps of Civilian Fire Fighters for service in Great Britain? Canada's answer was prompt. Yes – the Department of National War Services would recruit and organise a Corps of Fire Fighters on army lines and would maintain it in Britain.

To every fire department in Canada went the call for volunteers. The response was immediate. So the Corps was organised with men of long firefighting experience at the head.

Headquarters were set up on the top floor of an Ottawa fire station. Recruits began their special courses. At the beginning it may have seemed like kindergarten stuff to some of the men, for they were already trained from the ground up. But the courses were designed to bring them to new peaks of efficiency; to make them better firemen than they had been before. This was first-rate technical training along military lines.

Routines of physical training and basic military drill moulded the Corps into a fighting unit.

Use of the gas mask formed an important part of the training programme, because this was a danger that had to be taken into account when the men went overseas. They learned how to put on their respirators quickly even when on the march.

Familiar routines such as raising the heavy extension ladder were practised again. Even firemen of long experience found that their time improved with constant drills. They polished up and improved their firefighting techniques, practised with the useful short ladders.

Over and over again they went through the drill of working hose lines into buildings. They were given a thorough course in the use of life nets.

Quickly the Corps was whipped into shape, fighting fit and ready for battle. Soon they were overseas … the first firemen who ever answered a trans-ocean alarm. By Nelson's Monument, in the shade of Canada House in Trafalgar Square, they were given a royal welcome by the people of Britain.

Canadian firemen, reinforcements from abroad, ready to fight shoulder to shoulder with the hard-pressed smoke eaters of Britain.

The High Commissioner for Canada, Vincent Massey, was there and Home Secretary Herbert Morrison welcomed them to England. The Corps came under the administration of the Home Office, which directed the National Fire Services of Britain.

Crews were posted at once to four of the hottest areas under Blitz attacks, the big ports of Bristol, Portsmouth, Southampton and Plymouth, major targets of the Luftwaffe's fire bombs.

The men were often quartered in hospitable British homes, but in some areas they built their own stations.

And the training went on. Because now they had to master British firefighting equipment, some of it newly devised to cope with the special problems of the Blitz. These lessons had to be learned quickly.

They learned how to handle the 24 lb hook ladder with which a fireman can literally pull himself up by his own bootstraps from floor to floor of any building. Specially constructed mock-ups at the training stations were used for these practice drills. Even if a man had regarded himself as an expert fireman before he left Canada, he soon found his speed and timing improved. And if all this routine may have seemed dull at times, the men knew that these were skills upon which lives would depend.

Practice with the ladders constituted only one part of the programme. They were given very thorough training in the use of the foam extinguishers that had been developed as the most effective weapons against oil fires. British supplies of gas and oil were under constant attack by the Nazis. German bombers made repeated raids on dock areas to get at the oil storage tanks. The resulting fires were not only destructive, consuming great quantities of precious oil, but they were difficult to fight. The firemen learned how to use pourers fastened to the tops of extension ladders to get the foam into the burning tanks. They used their own drill tower for practice. This sort of drill was at least a good deal cooler than the real thing. As part of the programme, the firemen learned how to use the trailer pumps that had proven of special value in fighting oil fires. There were two types of foam inductors – in-line and portable models. They pumped up water from canvas tanks, and when foam compound was added to the inductor, a smothering stream was sent into the blazing oil. The men learned how to operate the handy valves that varied the foam and water mixture.

To master the technique of fighting oil fires also called for drill in the use of sprays. Often when oil fires could not be extinguished they could at least be kept from spreading. By using flat fan-tailed nozzles, the firemen were able to throw thin high walls of spray between the oil tanks. All this training was destined to play a big part in the fight to save Britain's vital oil supplies. In England, connections to the water supply are made below pavement level. The Canadian firemen were shown how to plug a connector into a pipe valve set in the water main. They were shown how to use devices that snapped the fittings into place in a matter of seconds.

Underground water mains, damaged by bomb blasts, were hard to get at and difficult to repair. Steel water pipes above ground provided one answer to the problem.

Sometimes the Canadian firemen ran up against peculiar water hydrant systems. In a few communities the main water pipe was equipped with wooden plugs. These would have to be knocked out to insert the wedge-shaped base of a portable hydrant. It was always a moist operation. [This is a rare moment of humour in the film, where we see the firefighters getting soaked as they attempt this operation.]

The Canadian Corps were well equipped. The men were particularly fond of their mobile kitchen.

Wartime first aid and training in rescue work from wrecked buildings formed an important part of the curriculum. All this training was essential before the men were ready for big-scale action. The fires were the pay-off. Here was the real test of the training plan that had started in Canada many months before. Lectures, drill and constant practice had shaped up a firefighting corps that knew its stuff.

And when they went into action they met the test not only as firefighters but as men. Smoke, heat, danger, long hours of gruelling work, these were the things they had been trained to face and to take in their stride. Many times they fought until they were overcome by smoke or exhaustion.

So the battle went on through the worst months of the Blitz [the worst months of the Blitz had passed by 1942, yet heavy raids continued, and the Canadians experienced firefighting and rescue work no less dramatic, especially during the V1 and V2 attacks], day after day, night after night, a discouraging and seemingly endless struggle. Often they had to give ground, but every fire was fought to the last spark and ember.

Daylight usually brought relief, and when the bombers had gone the people would come out of their shelters to gaze at their ruined shops and homes, to help clean up the rubble and to carry on somehow.

Slowly, steadily, Britain's aerial defence system became stronger. The raids became less violent and less frequent. In their spare time the Canadians supplemented their training with an active sports programme. Field days brought men of different detachments together.

Some of the field day events might have seemed strange to outsiders. But they were games and competitions that grew out of the work and out of the training programme. The winner of the hose rolling test knew the pride of a man who has proven himself good at his trade.

High points of the field day events was always the large trailer pump competitions. It always provided rivalry between fire force areas and between stations. It called for speed plus efficiency. Not only was the exercise run against time, but every part of every man's job was checked by expert judges. Any lapse meant that the crew's total time was increased by a penalty of seconds.

Teams in the trailer pump competition had to run out two lines of hose of two lengths each, connect the pump to the water tank, knock down the two standing targets, pick up and return the hoses to the trunk, then drive to the finish line. Teamwork really counts in this sort of race. And the teams knew that they were competing for something more than a silver cup. They were proving their ability to save seconds, seconds that might mean the saving of lives and property when the chips were down.

Before the Nazis folded up, they lashed out at Britain with new weapons, new methods of attack from the air. The island rocked and smoked to the onslaughts of the hit and run bombers, the robot bombs V1 and V2. Trained in the hard, tough school of the earlier Blitz fighting, the men of the Canadian Corps of Civilian Firefighters met these new threats with grim confidence. They fought beside their British comrades with courage and determination. When entire city blocks were burning it sometime seemed to civilians that the firemen were waging a hopeless battle. But each man's job fitted into a skilfully planned campaign. If big fires couldn't be put out, at least they could be kept from spreading.

Wherever the flames were the hottest, wherever smoke was the thickest, the Canadians upheld Canada's best traditions, the traditions of the fighting forces. Canadian firemen had gone to war as fighters, as firemen, as men. Men who have earned the respect and gratitude of Great Britain, men in whom all Canada takes pride.

In early 1946, the producer wrote the following letter to the National Film Board of Canada's UK office, care of the High Commission based in London:

Miss Kay Gillespie   Ottawa, Ontario
National Film Board of Canada   May 22, 1946
c/o High Commission for Canada
Canada House
London

Dear Kay
Greetings from the banks of the Ottawa all fresh and green and sultry (storms coming up)
Yesterday we shipped in your care –
1 Box containing 2 reels of B & W Silent Print 16mm
    "   2 reels of negative 16 mm
Subject – Firemen Go To War. Canadian Corps of Civilian Fire Fighters in the UK

These four reels are to be delivered to Mr N G Good, National Fire Services, Home Office, London, England
Here is the story briefly: Dept. of National War Service had on its overseas strength, during war one Company Officer Bruce Young who was equipped with a movie camera and supplied with Kodachrome film to keep a filmed record of the CCFF in

the UK. The unedited footage was given to me last year and with pain and protest we produced a two reel film out of the not so brilliantly shot footage.

Meanwhile – a request had come from Mr Good of the National Fire Service for whatever footage could be made available of the Canadians for inclusion in a film record of the national Fire Service. I understand the request was for 35mm Black and White. After further discussion we decided to send over a 16 mm B & W Negative taken from the Kodachrome original and for cutting purposes we are also supplying a Black and White print taken from the negative. We are not at all happy over the prospect of this footage – or whatever is selected – being blown up to 35mm and looking like anything on earth. But this is the only Canadian Footage available anywhere (we understand) and such as it is we are supplying it freely.

W A Macdonald

On the same day, the following letter was dispatched to the Home Office in London:

N G Good Esq.   Ottawa, Ontario
National Fire Service   May 22, 1946
Home Office
London, England

Dear Sir

Quite some time ago, Mr Chester Payne, Deputy Minister of National War Services for Canada, asked us on your behalf, to supply the best possible footage available of motion picture film showing members of the Canadian Corps of Civilian Fire Fighters in action in the United Kingdom.

At the time of Mr Payne's request we were editing some original Kodachrome footage supplied us by the photographic division of the Canadian Corps. Much of the footage was duplicative and not a little was poorly shot due to adverse conditions of location, weather and time. We have completed our editing of a two reel film and have been able to secure the footage you require only this week.

We understand from Mr Payne that you wanted footage to be considered for a film you were producing in 35 mm Black and White. We have 16 mm Kodachrome footage only. We are not happy about the probable result of the appearance of a 35 mm Black and White made from a 16 mm Kodachrome Original nor do we suppose you are very pleased with the prospect either. However, we have had a 16 mm Black and White print and a 16 mm Negative made for you.

We have today shipped the 4 reels (2 reels black and white and 2 reels negative) to Miss Kay Gillespie, National Film Board representative c/o High Commissioner for Canada, Canada House, London, England. This film is going forward by fast boat and Miss Gillespie will hand it over to you immediately she receives it. The film reaches you without cost but with the compliments of Mr Chester Payne, deputy Minister of national War services, Parliament Buildings, Ottawa, Canada. We hope you can make use of some of the footage and that your film production is completely successful

Very truly yours
W A Macdonald
Producer

The information sheet issued about the film on its official release in June 1946 states that:

Contents: The work done overseas by the Canadian Corps of Firefighters.

When the Battle of Britain was at its height, the British government appealed to the Canadian government for reinforcements for its National Fire Service. Recruiting began on a voluntary basis immediately and a corps was organised along military lines. The film gives details of the training received by members of the corps before proceeding overseas.

In Britain they were assigned to stations in cities the worst hit by the Blitz – Bristol, Southampton, Portsmouth and Plymouth. Here they learned new techniques of firefighting and learned to operate British equipment. The film shows us some of the rigid training which the corps underwent to fit it for its work. There are also scenes which show how the fire fighters occupied their spare time. There was a sports day for instance, but it is worth noting that many of the competitions grew out of the work which they performed every day.

When the Canadian firemen went into action they upheld the best traditions of Canadians in every branch of the armed services.

Canada subsequently embodied the experience gained by the Corps of Canadian Firefighters to help shape the provision of its peacetime Fire Service.

A British wartime fireman recorded:

I have the greatest admiration for the Corps of Canadian Fire Fighters. These men volunteered to leave the security and comfort of their homeland, face a perilous journey across the U-boat infested ocean and if they survived that journey, then faced an unknown period of danger, discomfort, short rations, uncomfortable living conditions and the possibility of becoming another entry in the Civilian War Dead Register.

Gentlemen, I salute you.

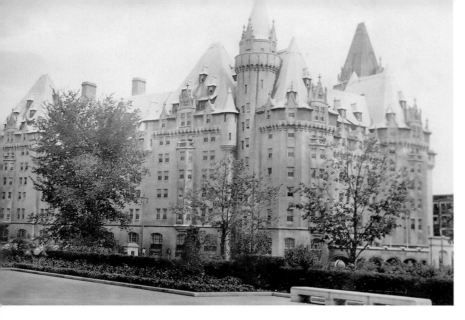

State Capital Building Ottawa
Left: The State Capital Building, photographed at the time of discussions about the formation of a volunteer Canadian fire force.

Government Building Ottawa
Right: One of several government buildings used for meetings about the formation of the volunteer fire force.

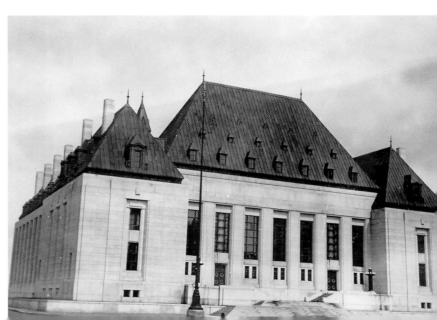

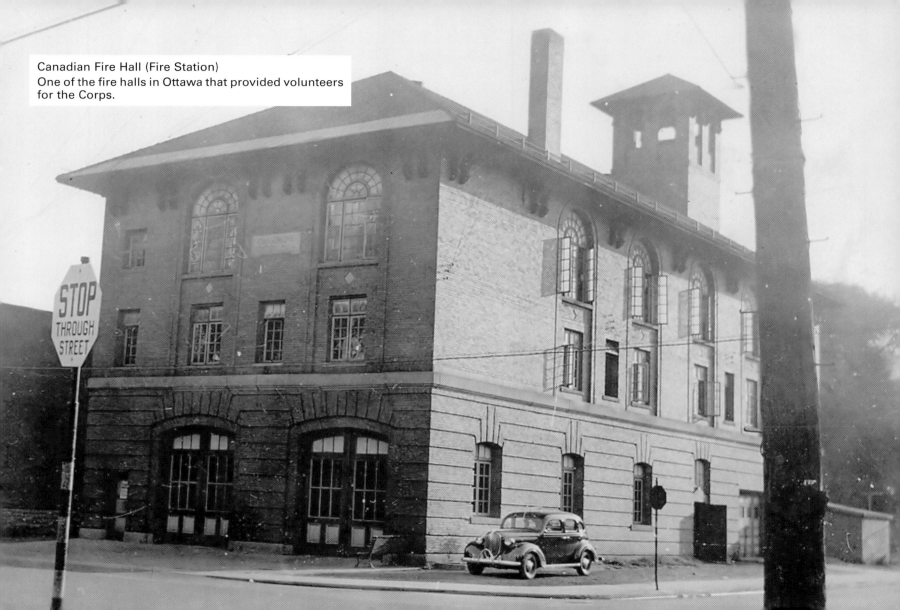

Canadian Fire Hall (Fire Station)
One of the fire halls in Ottawa that provided volunteers for the Corps.

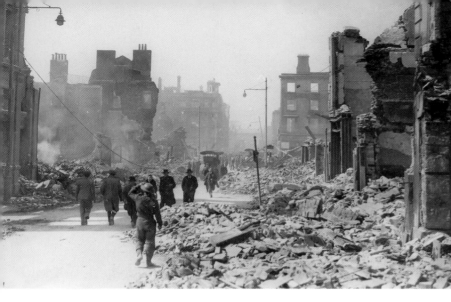

Plymouth II
Left: Plymouth after a raid, 1942.

Plymouth III
Right: Firefighters reported that the raid left very few houses as more than one storey in height.

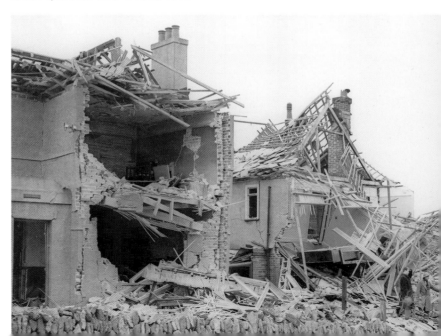

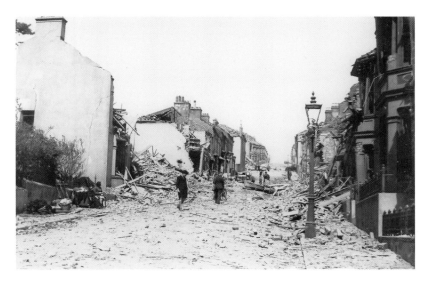

Personal Photos
Right: A group of eight personal photographs, which show injuries to one fire officer, sundry firefighting scenes and a parade.

Left: Plymouth During The War

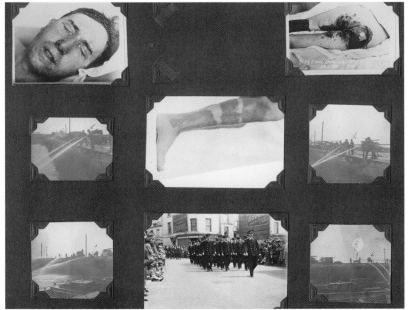

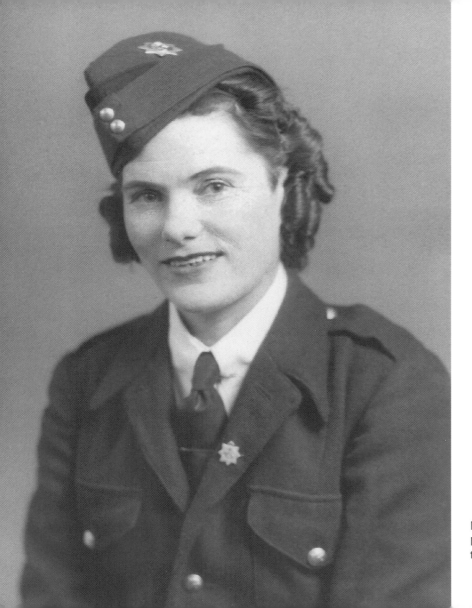

NFS Firewoman
May (Mary) Belbin was a firewoman at Testwood where the Canadians trained. She served refreshments when the service had field days.

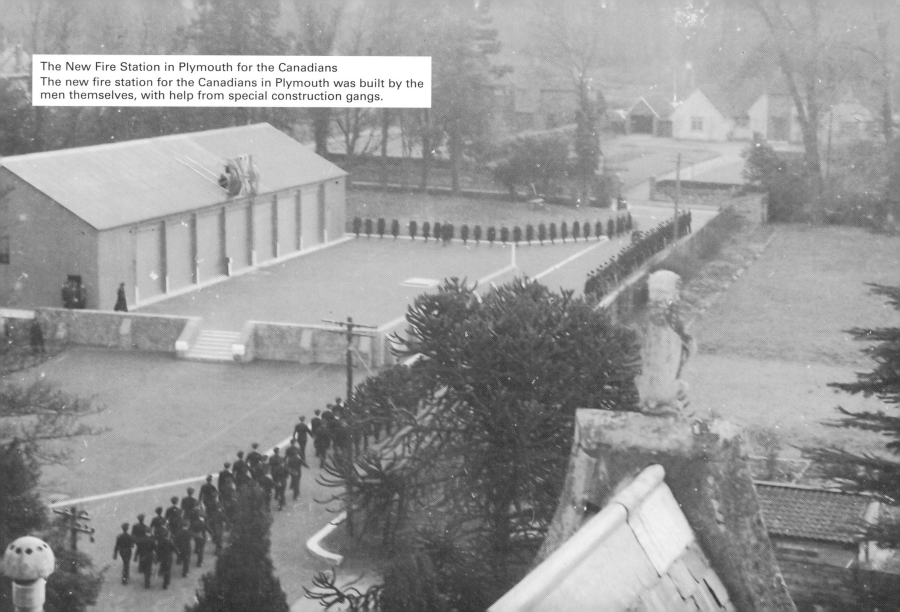

The New Fire Station in Plymouth for the Canadians
The new fire station for the Canadians in Plymouth was built by the men themselves, with help from special construction gangs.

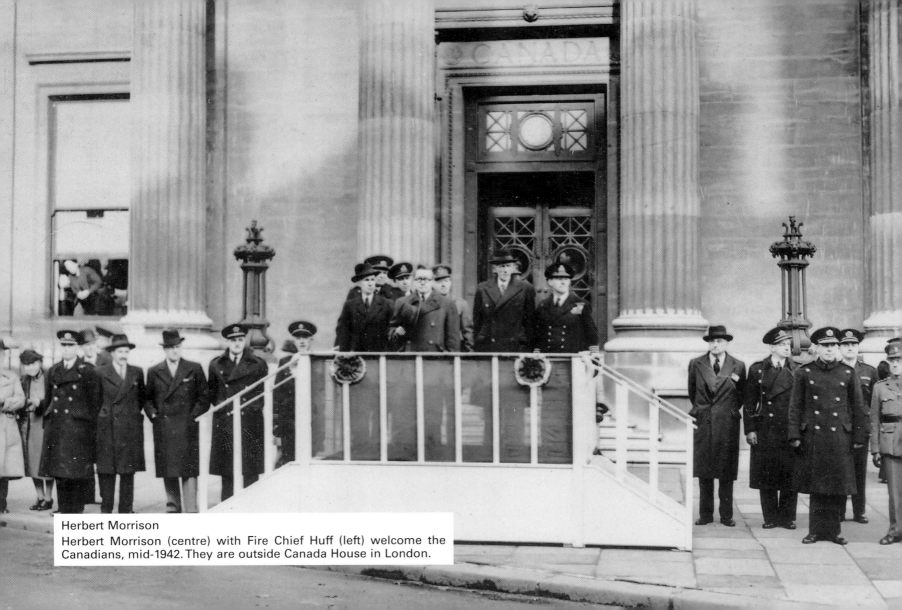

Herbert Morrison
Herbert Morrison (centre) with Fire Chief Huff (left) welcome the Canadians, mid-1942. They are outside Canada House in London.

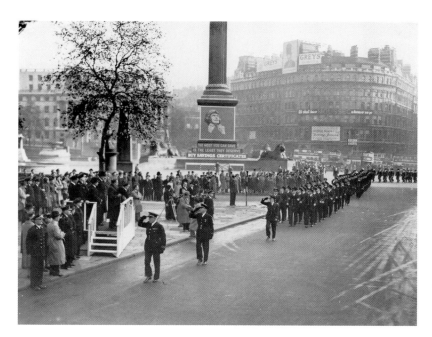

The Corps of Canadian Firefighters Arrive

Left: After two years of negotiations, the first Corps of Canadian Firefighters volunteers arrive in England.

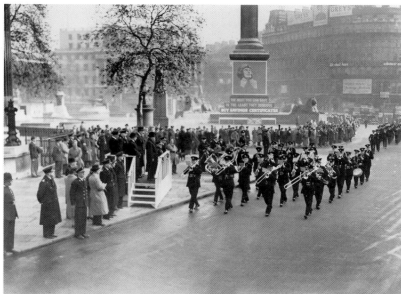

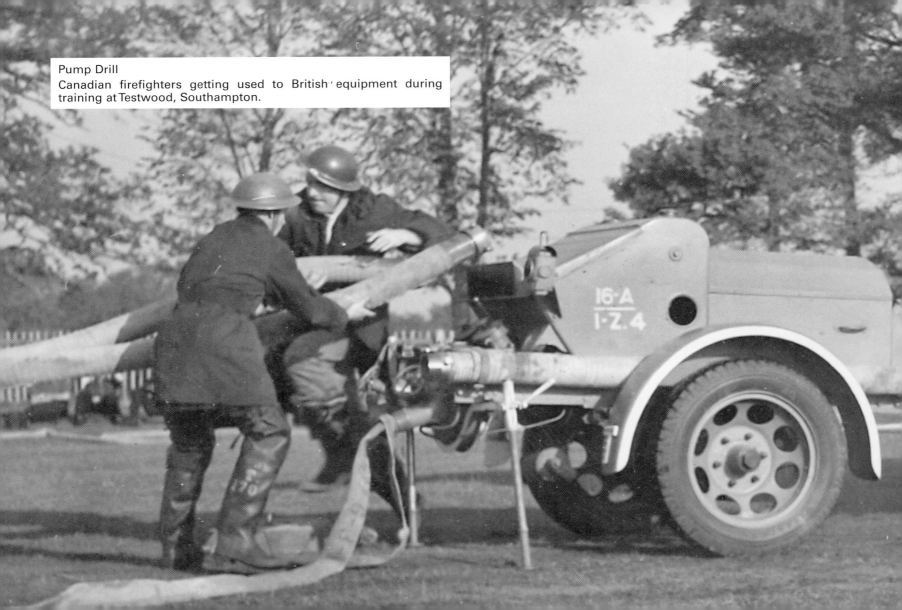

Pump Drill
Canadian firefighters getting used to British equipment during training at Testwood, Southampton.

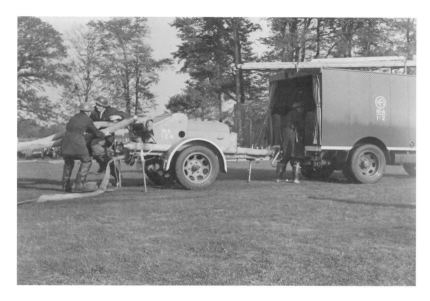

Pump Drill
Above: Training at Testwood, Southampton, this is for pump drill.

Duplicate
Right: All firefighters had to undergo tower training.

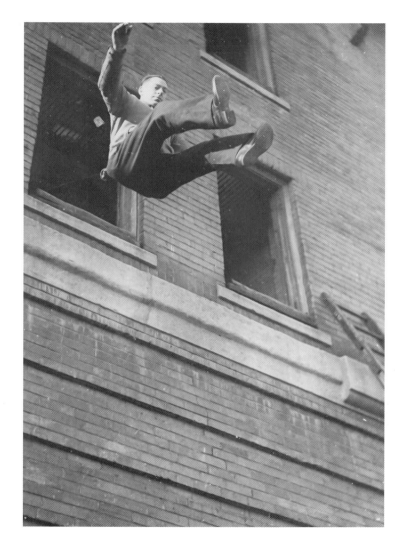

EPILOGUE

THE FIREMAN'S PRAYER

When I am called to duty, God
Whenever flames may rage
Give me the strength to save some life
Whatever be its age
Help me embrace the little child, before it is too late
Or save the older person from the horror of that fate
Enable me to be alert and hear the weakest shout
And quickly and efficiently to put the fire out
I want to fill my calling
And give the best in me
To guard my every neighbour and protect his property
And if according to your will I have to lose my life
Please bless with your protecting hands
My children and my wife.

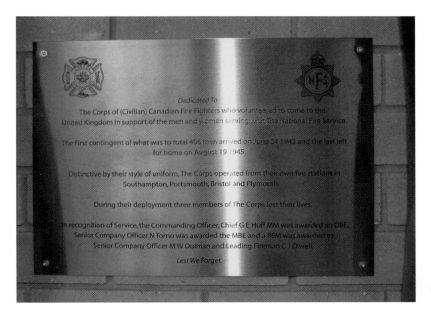

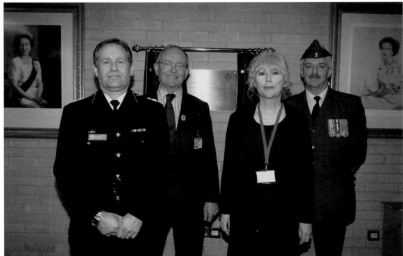

Left: The plaque dedicated to the CCFF at Eastleigh, Hampshire.

Right: Fire Officer House, Elaine Bryce (a relation of two of the CCFF members) and other guests at the unveiling ceremony.

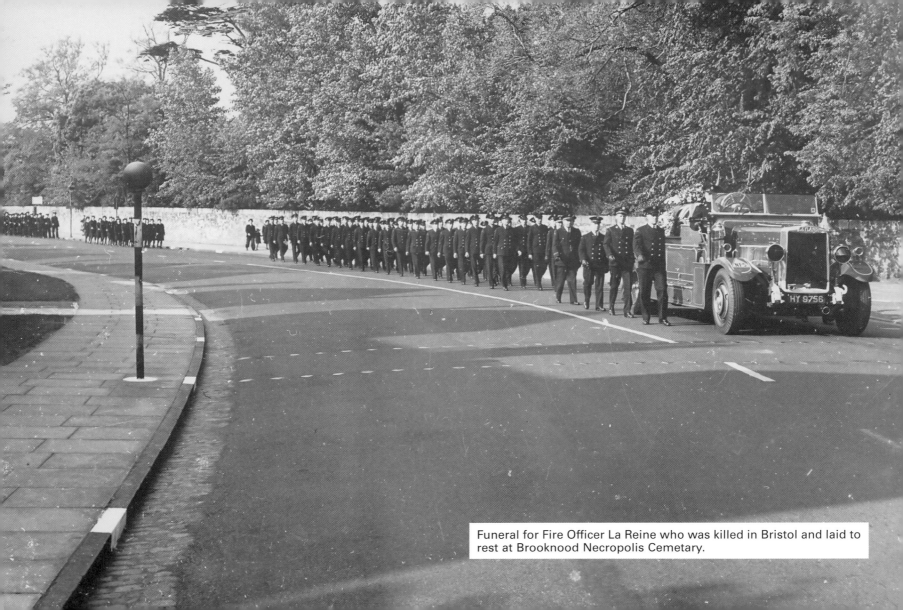

Funeral for Fire Officer La Reine who was killed in Bristol and laid to rest at Brooknood Necropolis Cemetary.

THE ETERNAL FLAME

In 1940 an unknown diarist wrote: 'The majority of people in Britain by the time the war came believed we were going to be bombed out of existence with incendiaries and personal bombs and gas.'

Fire is all-powerful and all-consuming. It provides heat and light and helps to sustain life, yet in contrast it can in a matter of seconds take life and cause destruction and devastation. It is a brave person who tackles fire head on. In the early days of the war firemen were subjected to taunts of draft-dodging, and these taunts continued until the 'baptism of fire' resulting from the Blitz in London and upon other cities in the country. Only then was the unquestionable value of the firefighting services and the men themselves proved beyond doubt.

The experience of wartime firefighters was taken to the wider British public in two films: an Ealing Studios feature film and one produced by the Crown Film Unit. Curiously both were released in April 1943. In their own way each was considered a classic piece of documentary, although only *The Bells Go Down*, starring Tommy Trinder and James Mason, had a storyline and a script.

Set in the East End of London, this ninety-minute film followed the experiences of a mixed group of AFS volunteers, and how they and the neighbourhood dealt with the challenges of the Blitz. Against this scenario, the crook (played by Mervyn Johns) rescues the policeman who before the war had arrested him. Tommy Tuck, the 'lovable' main character, played by Tommy Trinder, dies heroically trying to save the life of his hated commander.

In contrast the film *Fires Were Started*, running at just sixty-four minutes, had no script as such and the actors were all seconded NFS firemen. It records the lives and courage of seven firemen over a twenty-four-hour period, starting with the unit gathering at the fire station, preparing their equipment and taking part in training. They inspect the results of daytime bomb damage before getting together to socialise at the end of the day. A night-time raid is signalled by the siren, and the sound of anti-aircraft signals as the raid begins. Almost immediately the unit is called out to a warehouse upon which incendiaries have fallen, and the film follows the unit as they battle the blaze throughout the night. Since the war this film has been regarded by some as a particularly poignant kind of propaganda, although a fireman who watched the film on its release was not of the same opinion. In a diary entry made at the time, the unnamed writer recorded:

We went to see the film. It was a crazy mix up of AFS with NFS. A scene in the blitz of 1940/41 with IB's and HE's whamming down in a dock area and yet the girls are not wearing their tin hats!!! They are just hanging on the wall at the back. Girl on canteen van has no tin hat with her, hair all beautifully fluffed out as though she had just come out of the hairdressers. Oh yeah!

THE HUMAN COST

Mark Talbot remembers,

When it became apparent that the country was now likely to be bombed, all premises had to arrange for members of their staff to fire watch at night. In the city [London] some of the staff who lived in the suburbs and who had enough money, used to pay off-duty firemen to do their shifts for them.

The tonnage of bombs, flying bombs and rockets falling on the British Isles as recorded from 3 September 1939 to 8 May 1945 was 71.270. During the heavy raids on major cities from September 1940 to May 1941 approximately forty tons of bombs were dropped, with London taking the brunt of over eighteen thousand tons. By comparison, Manchester suffered

three attacks when just under six hundred tons were dropped, while Newcastle suffered 152 tons and Cardiff 115 tons.

Cyril Kendall recalls,

I remember when he (the enemy) dropped a stick of bombs down Queen Victoria Street in London In fact there is a very famous photograph of it. All the buildings along one side of the street toppled over like cards one after the other. We lost a lot of men and about fourteen machines that night. Luckily my crew were safe and we got away unscathed. Terrible, terrible incident.

In Britain, there were over 60,000 civilians killed and just over 86,000 injured as a result of enemy bombing. The peak strength of the Civil Defence Service including the Fire and Police Services was 1,869,000 thousand, although by 1945 this had dropped to just 359,000. The cost of maintaining the service from 1939 to 1946 was £983,430,000, a staggering figure, which today would top many billions of pounds.

Leading Fireman Wally Scott recalled the dangers of public shelters: 'For instance if a brick-built shelter was near enough to a bomb blast, the bricks would be blown away and would allow the concrete roof to fall on the occupants.' A vivid note in the diary of a witness brings home the personal cost: 'You can never forget the odour of burnt flesh. We had tears after every air raid. Even the men were visibly tearful.'

Nationally, 1,003 men and women serving with the Fire Service died as a result of enemy action while on duty, while 9,000 personnel were injured. Some 700 individual awards were made, including twenty-seven MBEs, two George Crosses and 187 British Empire Medals. The men and women of the fire services in the twenty-first century continue the tradition and spirit of their wartime counterparts, and continue to keep the eternal flame of remembrance burning.

In dogged mood the NFS awaits each night's alarms
Its men and women glory in the comradeship of arms
They've still their sense of humour, their ardour does not tire
In the service of the nation, for the mastery of fire

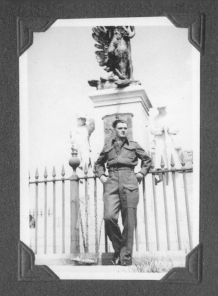

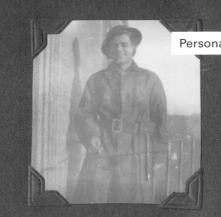

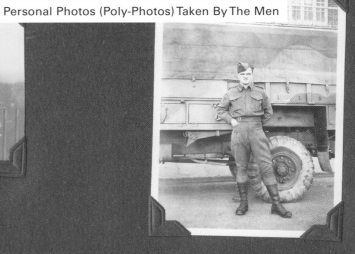

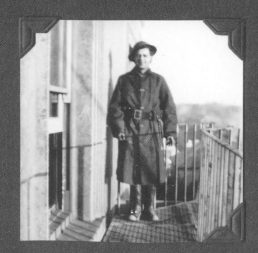

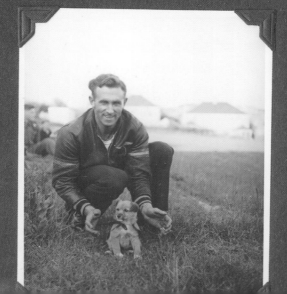

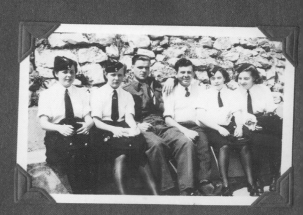

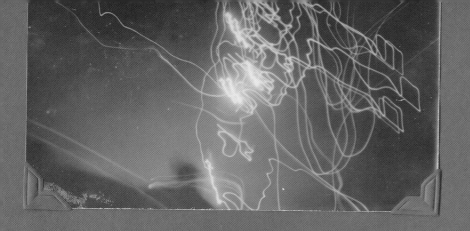

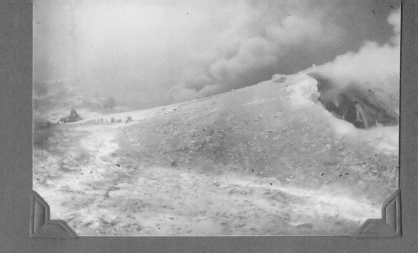

Personal Photos (Poly-Photos) Taken By The Men

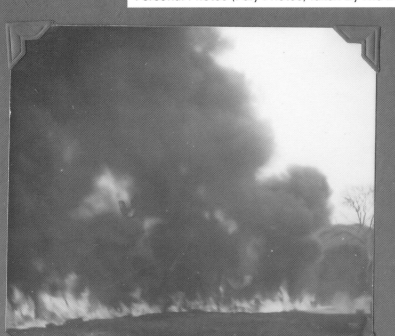

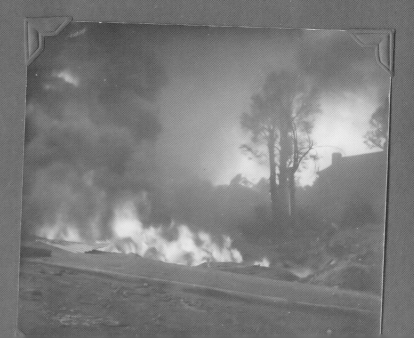

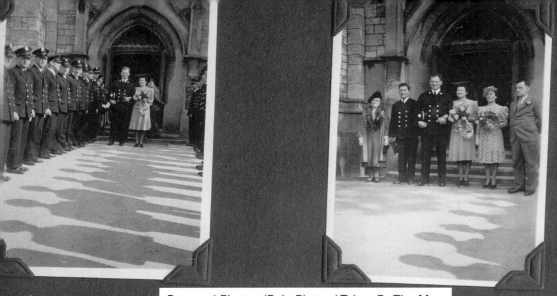

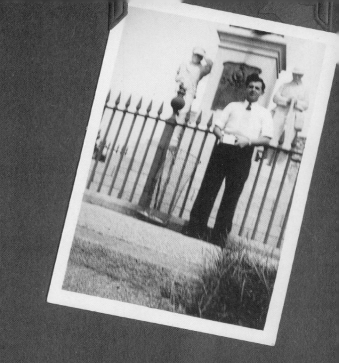

Personal Photos (Poly-Photos) Taken By The Men

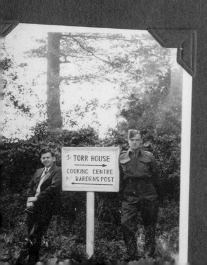

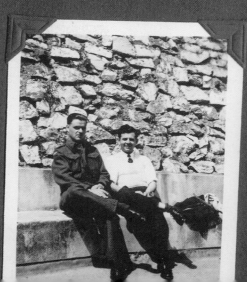

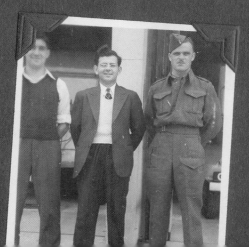

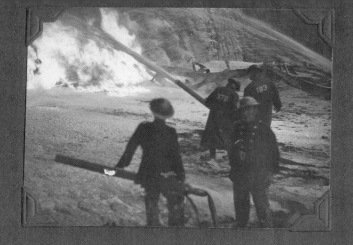

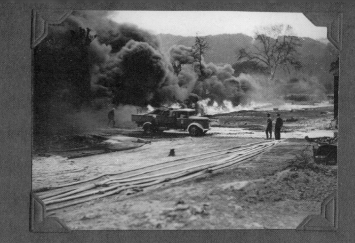

Personal Photos (Poly-Photos) Taken By The Men

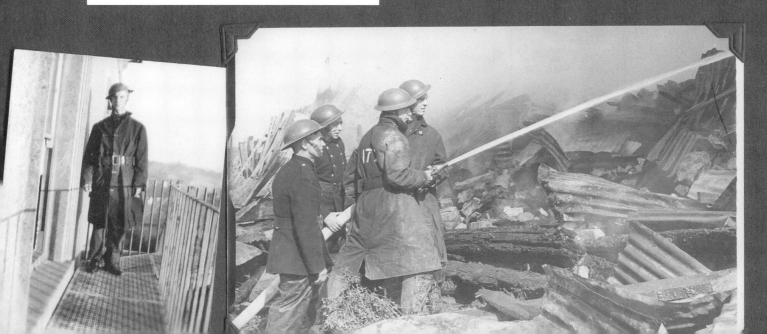

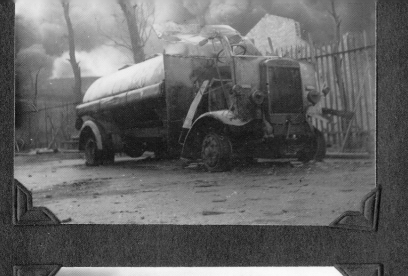

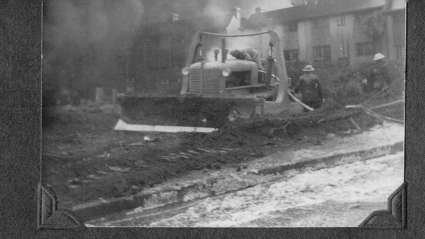

Personal Photos (Poly-Photos) Taken By The Men

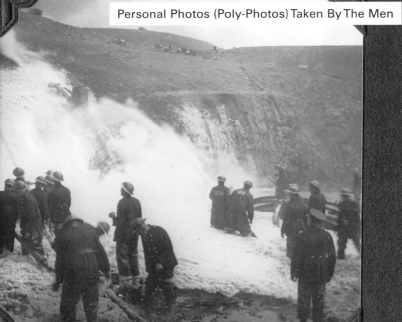

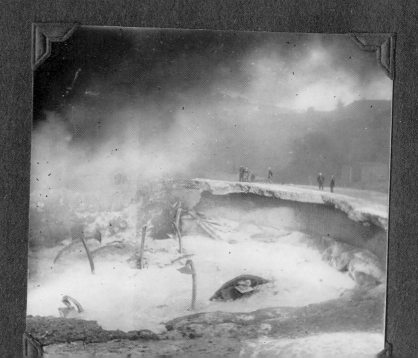

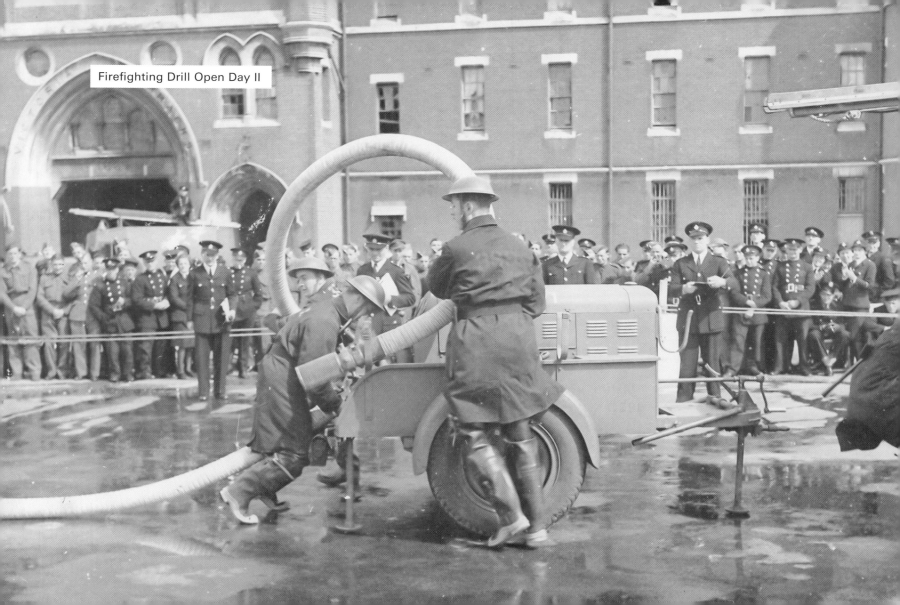

Firefighting Drill Open Day II

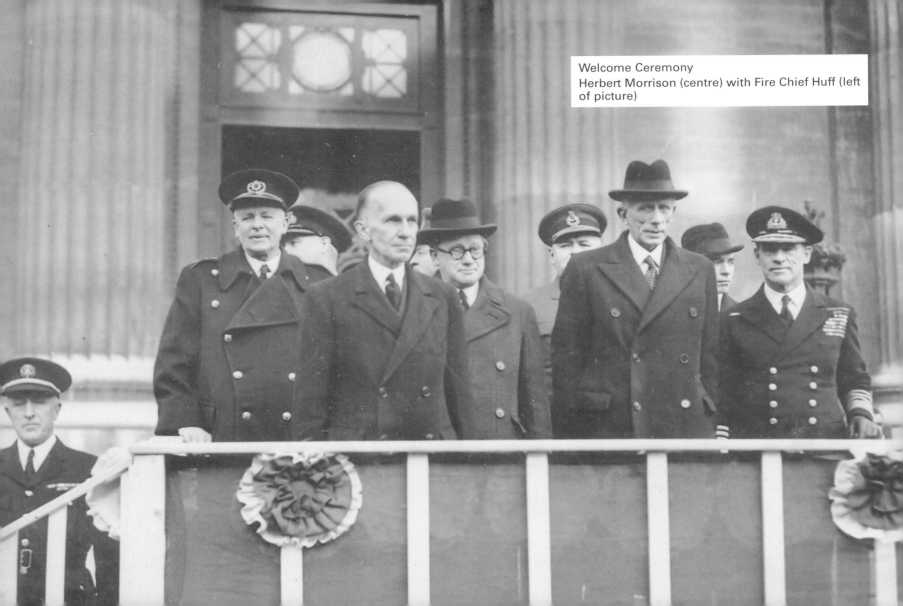

Welcome Ceremony
Herbert Morrison (centre) with Fire Chief Huff (left of picture)

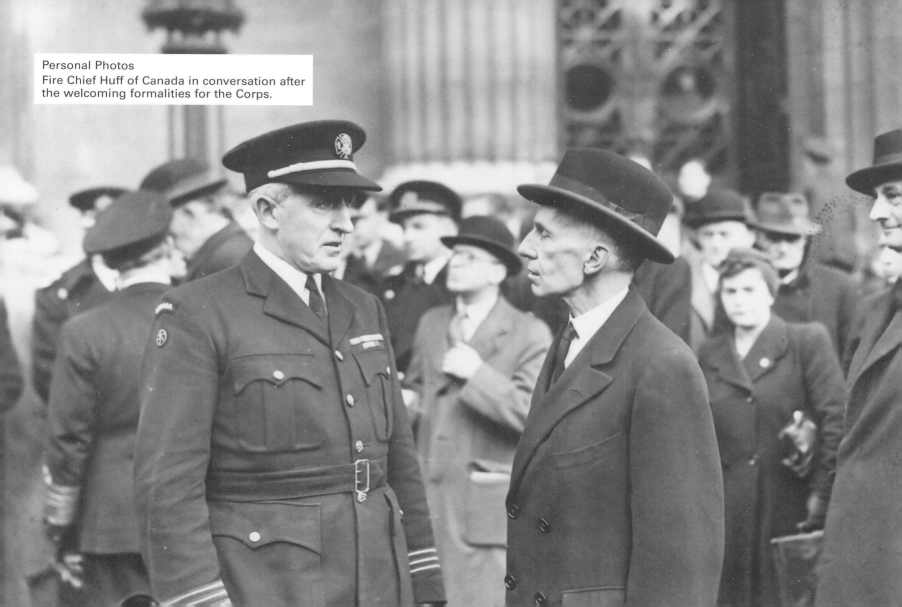

Fire Chief Huff of Canada in conversation after the welcoming formalities for the Corps.

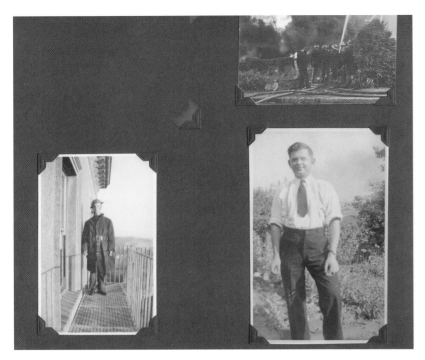

Personal Photos

Right and above: A selection of personal keepsake photographs of Corps members.

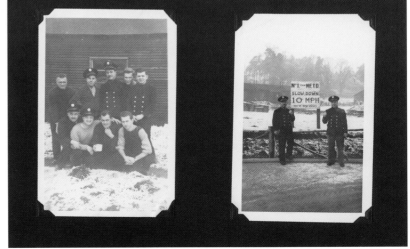

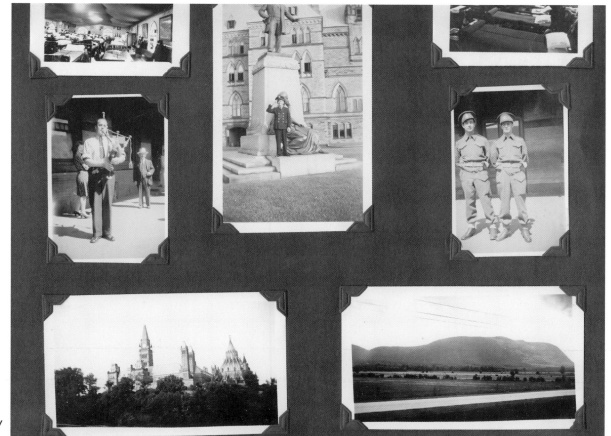

A Further Selection of Personal Photographs

Right and above: Members of the Corps were able to take photographs, as there appeared to be no problems regarding the supply of film.

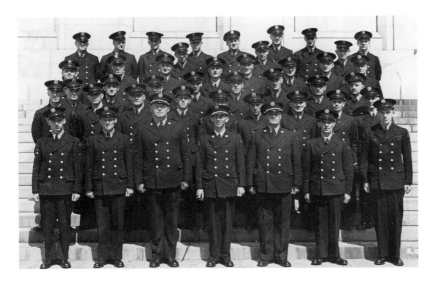

Fire Service Camp
Right: The Bristol and Plymouth contingents training centre at Ivy bridge, Devon.

Bristol 1942
Left: Some of the volunteers pictured just before leaving Canada.

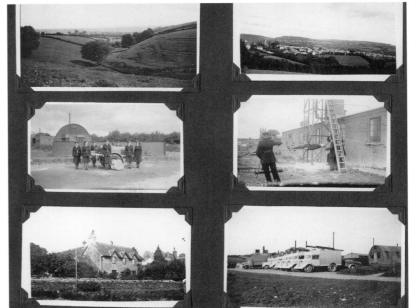

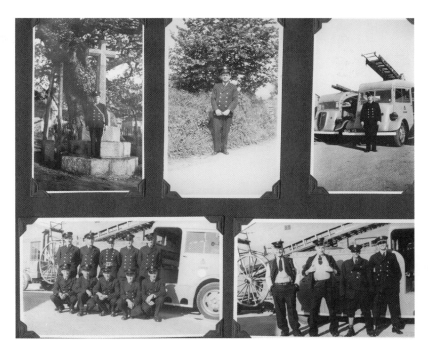

Above and right: Personal Photos

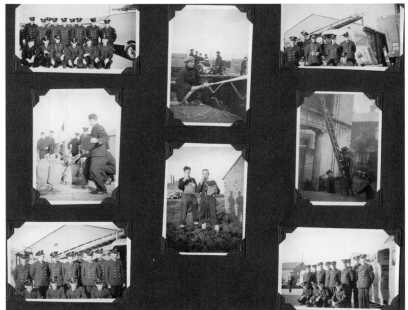

A new fire appliance with turntable ladder and pump comes in to service.

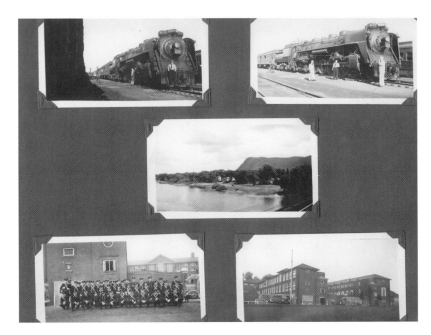

Right: Personal Photos.

Left: Some of the volunteers just before leaving Ottawa.

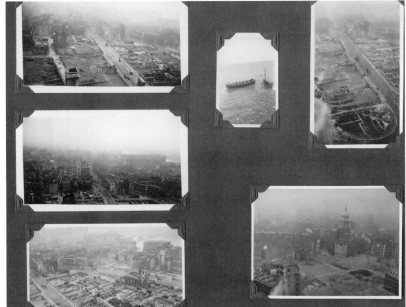

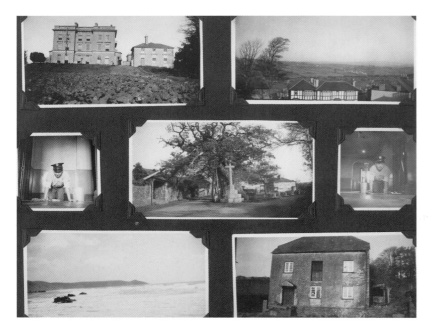

Right and above: Personal Photos

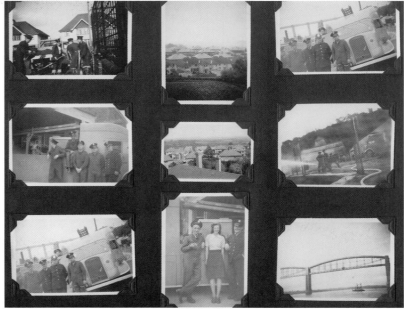

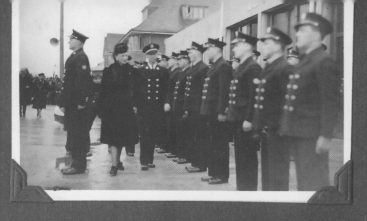

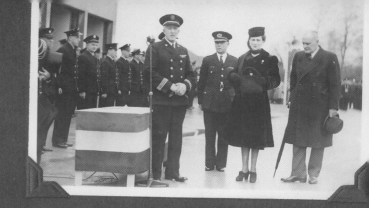

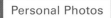
Personal Photos

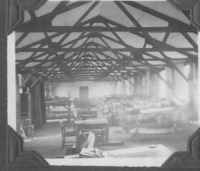

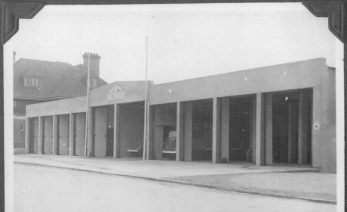

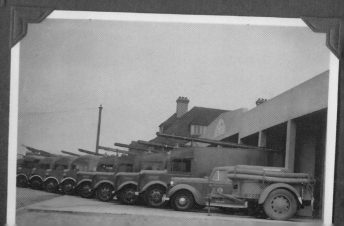

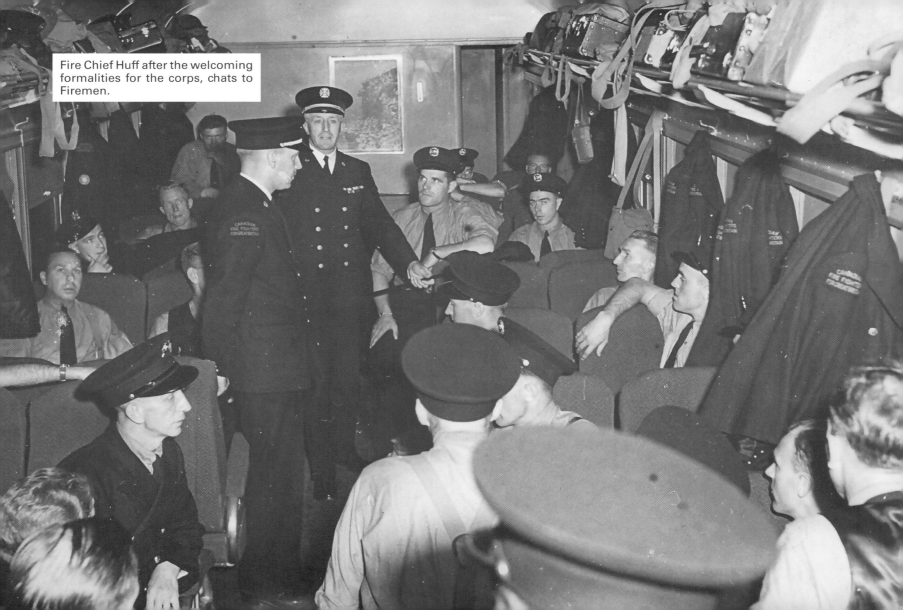

Fire Chief Huff after the welcoming formalities for the corps, chats to Firemen.

ACKNOWLEDGEMENTS

The authors would like to thank the following, without whose assistance this work would not have been possible:

Margaret Sheddon

Sir Graham Meldrum

Paul Landry

Simon Fletcher

Tom Gillmore

Ken Hampton

Tom Porter and family

May Belbin and family

Jack Coulter

Joyce Lewis

Cyril Kendall

Tom Adams

Phyllis Wilshaw

Dennis Perrett

Reginald Weekes

Ruth Davies

Davina Stevens

The Government of Canada

Canadian Police Department

National Film Board of Canada

Also Available from Amberley Publishing

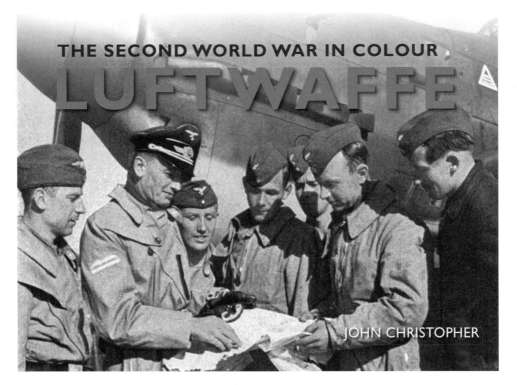

THE SECOND WORLD WAR IN COLOUR
LUFTWAFFE

JOHN CHRISTOPHER